Effective Sexual Health Interventions: Issues in experimental evaluation

Edited by

Judith M. Stephenson
Department of Sexually Transmitted Diseases
Royal Free and UCL Medical School
London

John Imrie
Department of Sexually Transmitted Diseases
Royal Free and UCL Medical School
London

Chris Bonell
Social Sciences Research Unit
Institute of Education
University of London

OXFORD
UNIVERSITY PRESS

OXFORD

UNIVERSITY PRESS

Great Clarendon Street, Oxford OX2 6DP

Oxford University Press is a department of the University of Oxford.
It furthers the University's objective of excellence in research, scholarship,
and education by publishing worldwide in

Oxford New York

Auckland Bangkok Buenos Aires Cape Town Chennai
Dar es Salaam Delhi Hong Kong Istanbul Karachi Kolkata
Kuala Lumpur Madrid Melbourne Mexico City Mumbai Nairobi
São Paulo Shanghai Taipei Tokyo Toronto

Oxford is a registered trade mark of Oxford University Press
in the UK and in certain other countries

Published in the United States
by Oxford University Press Inc., New York

A catalogue record for this title is available from the British Library

Library of Congress Cataloging in Publication Data

(Data available)

ISBN 0 19 850849 2 (Hbk)

10 9 8 7 6 5 4 3 2 1

Typeset by Newgen Imaging Systems (P) Ltd, Chennai, India
Printed in Great Britain
on acid-free paper by
T.J. International Ltd, Padstow, Cornwall

Foreword

In the mid-1960s, just before I was let loose on an unsuspecting British public as a qualified, inexperienced medical practitioner, I bought a copy of Dr. Benjamin Spock's best-selling book *'Baby and Child Care'*. At that time, this little book of advice for parents had sold over 19 million copies, making it the best-selling new title since best-seller lists began. I marked a passage in the book, which read: 'There are two disadvantages to a baby's sleeping on his back. If he vomits, he's more likely to choke on the vomitus. Also he tends to keep his head turned towards the same side...this may flatten the side of his head...I think it is preferable to accustom a baby to sleeping on his stomach from the start.' No doubt like millions of Spock's other readers, I passed on and acted on his apparently rational advice. We know now that the advice he promulgated so successfully in his seismic bestseller led to thousands, if not tens of thousands, of avoidable cot deaths.

This and other examples should be a sobering warning to those who promulgate health advice without ensuring that reliable empirical research evidence has shown that their prescriptions and proscriptions are more likely help than to harm other people. What do I mean by 'reliable empirical evidence'? Research using two types of observational data convinced me that I had done harm by promulgating Dr Spock's 'rational' advice. First, case-control studies convinced me that prone sleeping position was an independent risk factor for death during infancy. Second, the reduction in the incidence of cot deaths associated with the 'Back to Sleep Campaign' was so dramatic that I accepted it as strong evidence that Spock's advice, and my health education practice, had been tragically wrong.

It is very rare for health education to have effects as dramatic as the 'Back to Sleep Campaign'. Usually, the challenge is to identify moderate but important beneficial and adverse effects reliably, and to distinguish them from the influences of inadequately controlled biases. At the end of the day, causal inferences about the impact of health education on people's lives will require leaps of faith. It is because these leaps can result in unintended harm, however, that careful consideration of the evidential basis for them is so important. And because the results of randomized experiments differ in unpredictable ways from the results of non-randomized evaluations (1), methodological choices are inescapable. Thus, for example, non-randomized research suggests that educational programmes targeting teenagers with the intention of reducing road crashes are effective; whereas the only effect detected in randomized experiments of these programmes is that they induce teenagers to start driving at a younger age (2).

Although this book focuses on the use of randomized experiments in health education, most of the chapters stress the importance of methodological eclecticism: different methodological horses are appropriate for different methodological courses. One of the contributors, however, rejects randomized experiments completely, and her views are quite common among social scientists. My interest in research is motivated by a concern to minimize the unintended harm professionals (including health educators) do to other people. Our knowledge of the factors that influence health will always remain incomplete. Randomization helps to protect us from the adverse effects of this inevitable ignorance. Those who reject the only methodological feature specific to randomized experiments—randomization itself—strike me as recklessly arrogant. I hope that this book will encourage humility among practitioners and researchers about their capacity for doing harm, and will persuade them to make appropriate use of randomization to reduce biases from unmeasured but important determinants of health.

Iain Chalmers
James Lind Initiative

References

1. **Kunz, R., Vist, G., and Oxman, A.D.** (2002) Randomisation to protect against selection bias in healthcare trials (Cochrane Methodology Review). In: The Cochrane Library, Issue 4. Oxford: Update Software.
2. **Achara, S., Adeyemi, B., Dosekun, E., Kelleher, S., Lansley, M., Male, I., Muhialdin, N., Reynolds. L., Roberts, I., Smailbegovic, M., and van der Spek, N.** (2001) The Cochrane Injuries Group Driver Education Reviewers. Evidence based road safety: the Driving Standards Agency's schools programme. *Lancet,* **358**, 230–2.

Preface

In recent years, an international movement for evidence-based practice has developed. It aims to assess the effectiveness of health service, and other, interventions in order to inform judgements about which should continue to be provided, and which should be amended or dropped. Experimental methods are often championed as the most rigorous means of evaluating effectiveness. However, experimental evaluation remains controversial, especially in fields that mainly employ social and behavioural, as opposed to clinical, approaches, and in fields where a multitude of groups, with different views on what constitutes evidence, are engaged in evaluation.

This book aims to explore the philosophical, ethical, and methodological issues involved in the experimental evaluation of social and behavioural interventions. It focuses on sexual health as an example of the sort of field, described above, where controversy continues. The book considers the merits and limitations of randomized trials in evaluating sexual health interventions, and discusses what issues must be addressed in order to maximize the validity of experimental methods. We hope that this book contributes to improvements in the evaluation of social and behavioural interventions, both in the field of sexual health and elsewhere.

The book is intended to appeal both to those already convinced of the value of experimental evaluation, and to those with a more sceptical, but nonetheless curious, view of experimentation. The book considers the issues involved in experimental evaluation, rather than reporting the findings of particular experimental studies. It explores evaluation in both developed and developing countries. Although the book focuses on sexual health, we believe that most of the issues discussed are relevant to other fields of health and social policy where social and behavioural approaches are employed. We hope the book will be of interest to health service, and other medical and social, researchers, to health practitioners and managers, to health promotion and public health specialists, and to those training in, or otherwise studying, these disciplines.

The first section of the book addresses the question, to experiment or not? It explores why experimental evaluation of sexual health interventions is such a hotly contested issue, and considers whether than other health interventions: sexual health interventions are less amenable to experimental evaluation. Section two deals with more methodological issues. It examines the role that theory might play in the development and evaluation of interventions, and considers the relative merits of different randomized designs. Other chapters in this section consider what outcome measures are appropriate, and what other information needs to be collected within trials. The third section considers what happens after completion of sexual health trials. It explores how evaluation findings can be used to inform policy and practice, and to promote the use of effective and sustainable interventions. It examines the utility of systematic reviews and meta-analyses in summarizing the findings of multiple experimental studies of sexual health interventions. Drawing on the different contributions to this book, the final chapter considers the challenges facing behavioural intervention trials, and how to increase the utility of future trials in the pursuit of better sexual health.

Judith Stephenson
John Imrie
Chris Bonell

London 2002

Contents

Contributors

Rebecca Bennett
University of Manchester
Oxford Road
Manchester M13 9PL
UK

Sheila Bird
MRC Biostatistics Unit
Institute of Public Health
University of Cambridge
Robinson Way
Cambridge CB2 2SR
UK

Chris Bonell
Social Science Research Unit
Institute of Education
University of London
18 Woburn Square
London WC1H 0NS
UK

Jane Champion
University of Texas Health Science
  Centre at San Antonio
Department of Family Nursing
7703 Floyd Curl Drive
San Antonio, TX 78229-3900
USA

Frances Cowan
Department of Sexually Transmitted
  Diseases
Royal Free and University College
  Medical School
University College London
The Mortimer Market Centre
Off Capper Street
London WC1E 6AU
UK

Jonathan Elford
City University London
Institute of Health Sciences and
  St. Bartholomew School of Nursing
  and Midwifery
20 Bartholomew Close
London EC1A 7QN
UK

Heiner Grosskurth
Department of Infectious and
  Tropical Diseases
HIV/STI Prevention and Care
  Research Programme
The Population Council
142 Golf Links
New Delhi 110003
India

Angela Harden
EPPI Centre
Social Science Research
  Unit
Institute of Education
18 Woburn Square
London WC1H 0NR
UK

Graham Hart
MRC Social and Public
  Sciences Health Unit
University of Glasgow
6 Lilybank Gardens
Glasgow
G12 8RZ
UK

Richard Hayes
Department of Infectious and
  Tropical Diseases
London School of Hygiene and
  Tropical Medicine
Keppel Street
London WC1E 7HT
UK

Alan E. C. Holden
University of Texas Health Science
  Centre at San Antonio
Department of Obstetrics and
  Gynaecology
7703 Floyd Curl Drive
San Antonio, TX 78229-3900
USA

John Imrie
Department of Sexually
  Transmitted Diseases
Royal Free and University
  College Medical School
University College London
The Mortimer Market Centre
Off Capper Street
London WC1E 6AU
UK

Mary Kamb
Prevention Services Research Branch
Division of HIV / AIDS Prevention
MS E-46, Centres for Disease
  Control and Prevention
1600 Clifton Road NE
Atlanta, GE 20222
USA

Susan Kippax
National Centre in HIV Social
  Research
Sir Robert Webster Building – Level 2
University of New South Wales
Sydney NSW2052
Australia

Lilani Kumaranayake
Department of Public Health and
  Policy
London School of Hygiene and
  Tropical Medicine
Keppel Street
London WC1E 7HT
UK

Irwin Nazareth
Department of Primary Care and
  Population Sciences
Royal Free and University College
  Medical School
Rowland Hill Street
London NW3 2PF
UK

Edward R. Newton
Department of Obstetrics and
  Gynaecology
East Carolina University
School of Medicine
Room 162 PCMH Teaching
  Annex
Greenville, NC 27858-4354
USA

Ann Oakley
Social Science Research
  Unit
Institute of Education
University of London
18 Woburn Square
London WC1H 0NS
UK

Angela Obasi
London School of Hygiene and
  Tropical Medicine
Keppel Street
London WC1E 7HT
UK

Angela Obasi
African Medical Research
  Foundation
PO Box 2773
Dar es Salaam
Tanzania

Sondra T. Perdue
University of Texas Health Science
  Centre at San Antonio
Department of Microbiology
7703 Floyd Curl Drive
San Antonio, TX 78229-3900
USA

Jeanna M. Piper
University of Texas Health Science
  Centre at San Antonio
Department of Obstetrics and
  Gynaecology
7703 Floyd Curl Drive
San Antonio, TX 78229-3900
USA

Mary Plummer
Department of Infectious and
  Tropical Diseases
London School of Hygiene and
  Tropical Medicine
Keppel Street
London WC1E 7HT
UK

David Ross
Department of Infectious and
  Tropical Diseases
London School of Hygiene and
  Tropical Medicine
Keppel Street
London WC1E 7HT
UK

Rochelle Shain
University of Texas Health Science
  Centre at San Antonio
Department of Obstetrics and
  Gynaecology
7703 Floyd Curl Drive
San Antonio, TX 78229-3900
USA

Jonathan Shepherd
EPPI Centre
Social Science Research Unit
Institute of Education
18 Woburn Square
London WC1H 0NR
UK

Judith Stephenson
Department of Sexually Transmitted
  Diseases
Royal Free and University College
  Medical School
University College London
The Mortimer Market Centre
Off Capper Street
London WC1E 6AU
UK

Stephen Sutton
University of Cambridge
Institute of Public Health
Robinson Way
Cambridge CB2 2SR
UK

Daniel Wight
MRC Social and Public Health
  Sciences Unit
4 Lilybank Gardens
Glasgow
G12 8RZ
UK

Abbreviations

AB	Attitude towards behaviour
ACASI	Audio computer-assisted self-interviewing
AIDS	Acquired immunodeficiency syndrome
AMREF	African Medical and Research Foundation
ARHI	Adolescent reproductive health intervention
ARRM	AIDS risk reduction model
B	Behaviour
BB	Behavioural beliefs
BI	Behavioural intention
CEA	Cost-effectiveness analysis
CRTs	Cluster randomized trials
DALY	Disability adjusted life year
DoH	Department of Health
DSMBs	Data Safety Monitoring Boards
EIA	Enzyme linked immunoassay
ELISA	Enzyme linked immunosorbent assay
EPPI-Centre	Evidence Informed Policy and Practice Information and Coordination Centre
FGD	Focus Group discussions
GEE	Generalized estimating equations
GMTF	Gay Men's Task Force
GUM	Genitourinary medicine
HAART	Highly active antiretroviral therapy
HIV	Human immunodeficiency virus
HPV	Human papilloma virus
HSV-2	*Herpes Simplex* virus type 2
LE	Leukoesterase dipstick test
LSHTM	London School of Hygiene and Tropical Medicine
NB	Normative beliefs
NIMH	National Institute of Mental Health
OR	Odds ratio
RR	Relative risk
SD	Standard deviation
SHARE	Sexual Health and Relationships: Safe, Happy and Responsible Sex Education Programme
SN	Subjective norm

STD	Sexually transmitted diseases
STI	Sexually transmitted infection
TPB	Theory of planned behaviour
TRA	Theory of reasoned action

Section 1

To experiment or not

Why are randomised trials considered the method of choice for evaluating the effectiveness of interventions? Are sexual health interventions inherently unsuitable for experimental evaluation? Why is this such a hotly contested issue?

Chapter 1

Sexual health interventions should be subject to experimental evaluation

Chris Bonell, Rebecca Bennett, and
Ann Oakley

Introduction

The term 'sexual health intervention' can be applied to many different types of
treatment or other activity designed to improve sexual health. These include
medical interventions targeted at detecting and treating sexually transmitted
infections (STIs), as well as 'health promotion' interventions aimed primarily
at modifying sexual behaviour through effects on knowledge, attitudes, and
skills. The latter are the main focus of this book. Health promotion can involve
face-to-face communication, such as counselling or community outreach, or
mediated communication, such as television advertisements or posters.[1]

Caplan categorizes health promotion in terms of two dimensions. Firstly,
health promotion can aim to affect the actions of individuals, or to modify the
social environment or 'structure' within which individuals live.[2] For example,
sexual health promotion might, at an individual level, try to improve gay men's
self-esteem, and/or, at the structural level, try to challenge societal homophobia.
Secondly, health promotion can be driven by the priorities and views of affected
individuals, or by those of 'experts'. For example, health promotion in the area
of teenage pregnancy might be planned with active input from teenagers, or
professionals might direct it with no such input. In practice, most health promotion has been individual-focused and 'expert-driven'.[3] This is probably true
of sexual health promotion too, although, as discussed later, some interventions
have addressed the structural determinants of risk, and some interventions have
been planned with the involvement of affected communities.

Why should sexual health promotion be evaluated?

HIV/AIDS and other STIs and unintended pregnancies have extremely
important consequences for health. Policy-makers, practitioners, and affected

communities need to know whether sexual health interventions are effective in achieving key outcomes, such as reductions in rates of infections or unintended pregnancies, or perhaps changes in behaviours associated with reductions in these rates. Although it is necessary to examine process measures, such as whether affected communities participate in health promotion planning,[4] process measures are on their own insufficient. We need to know whether interventions do what they are meant to do. Effectiveness cannot be assumed: some sexual health promotion interventions have been shown to be ineffective.[5,6]

Evaluation is also needed to minimize the deployment of harmful interventions.[5] Although some may believe there to be little likelihood of health promotion (as opposed to pharmacological or surgical) interventions causing harm, this possibility is very real. For example, Christopher and Roosa[7] found greater sexual risk-taking among adolescent males subject to a school-based sexual abstinence programme than those in a comparison group. In a study of gay men attending a genitourinary (GUM) clinic,[8] the risk of STI was unexpectedly higher in men randomized to a small group intervention designed to reduce sexual risk behaviour than in the control group randomized to standard management. Oakley gives other examples of social interventions that were unexpectedly found to cause harm.[9]

Evaluation is also needed because, in the context of limited funding for health services, it is necessary to promote the most cost-effective array of interventions possible. This is particularly so with sexual health promotion because of the poor resourcing of this area nationally and globally.[10,11]

Evaluation is therefore important to: maximize deployment of effective interventions; stop harmful interventions being further deployed; and maximize the cost-effectiveness of interventions. Although the effectiveness of some sexual health promotion interventions has been evaluated,[5,12] in most cases it has not.

Why use experimental designs?

Experimental designs generally compare the baseline and outcome measures of one or more intervention groups (participants who are allocated to receive the interventions being evaluated) with those of one or more comparison groups (participants who are allocated to receive 'care as usual', which may be nothing at all or routinely available services). Non-experimental designs do not include a comparison group.

To evaluate the effectiveness of interventions rigorously, it is necessary to establish, with some confidence, an association between positive outcomes and exposure to the intervention in question. The possibility that such an association reflects the effect of some other factor should be minimised. In a non-experimental study, that is one that lacks a control group, an improvement in outcome measures compared with baseline measures might reflect the effect of the intervention or may indicate the confounding effect of some other change over time, such as secular trends or the effects of ageing of the cohort. In an experimental study, both intervention and control groups are subject to the same changes over time, which can therefore be distinguished from the effect of the intervention itself. Attributing differences in outcome between the two groups to the intervention also requires the two groups to be similar at baseline. Random allocation to intervention or control group is the best way to achieve this, and is discussed further in Chapter 3. Instead of using random allocation, some studies employ a matched control group. Randomized controlled trials are generally regarded as more rigorous than matched controlled trials because they afford greater control over bias.[13] The problem with matched studies is that, in order to match successfully, investigators need to know about all the relevant factors that can influence outcome, and this is unlikely to be the case. Randomization has the advantage that it should distribute factors that influence the outcome—both known an unknown—equally between intervention and comparison groups. It is thus an elegantly simple device for taking account of the multiplicity of social influences on outcomes studied in research.[14]

To provide useful data on effectiveness, experimental methods must be rigorously designed. This means they must employ outcome measures that are valid and reflect the aims of key stakeholders including the affected communities. They must also employ large enough samples to minimize the possibility that the play of chance, that is random error, could account for the findings. Criteria for establishing the rigour of an experimental evaluation commonly include reporting on baseline characteristics of the intervention and comparison groups, all the outcomes identified in the aims of the evaluation for both groups, and also attrition within each of these groups.[5,6] Randomized trials should describe how randomization was achieved, for example, by using random number tables, rather than merely being described as 'random'. These points are as true for the evaluation of sexual health promotion as for any other intervention.

The value of controlled trials is apparent when these are compared with other designs.[15] In a review of interventions for adolescent pregnancy prevention, observational studies compared with RCTs significantly overestimated intervention effectiveness.[16] Process evaluations have commonly been used to examine sexual health interventions.[17] These designs play an important role in evaluation, and, indeed, are the only way to assess the mode of operation of an intervention, as discussed further in Chapter 10. However, process evaluations alone cannot determine the *effectiveness* of interventions as rigorously as experimental studies, because they focus on how an intervention is delivered rather than its effects on participants.

Cohort studies have also been used to examine the effects of HIV prevention interventions.[18] In a cohort study, a group of people are defined at a point in time on the basis of their exposure or lack of exposure to some putative health determinant—which could be a health promotion intervention—and then followed up over time. As mentioned above, a cohort study without a control group of unexposed individuals can only provide weak evidence about the effects of an intervention. Besides age-related trends, participants might change their behaviour over time in response to other health promotion campaigns or to events portrayed in the media. Participants might even have received the sexual health promotion intervention in the first place because they were taking more risks than they normally would, and their behaviour then naturally settles down to its normal pattern afterwards, irrespective of the intervention.[19] Cohort designs are therefore not the most efficient ways of exploring the ways in which the intervention and other factors may interact in influencing sexual actions and health.

Ecological studies have also been used to examine the effectiveness of HIV prevention interventions.[20] These involve non-randomized and non-matched comparisons between populations rather than individuals; they cannot provide unbiased information on the effects of interventions, nor can they report on the influence of interventions on individuals, only on the apparent effects of interventions on whole populations.

Some researchers seems to suggest that all research designs are equally valid and what matters is how rigorously research is done.[21] It is true that all research designs are useful in answering some research question or other, and true that, to be of value, research must be conducted rigorously. However, it is not true that all research designs, if applied rigorously, are equally useful in answering *all* research questions.[15] Just as an experimental outcome evaluation, in itself, is of no value in examining process, a process evaluation is of no value in examining whether an intervention is effective. However, process evaluation can answer important questions about the factors influencing the development, provision and delivery of an intervention, and help to explain *why* something works or not. The key to good evaluation lies in using different designs appropriately.

Arguments against experimental evaluation

Ethical arguments

Some authors argue that it is unethical to evaluate sexual health promotion interventions by means of randomized trials because participants in control groups are deprived of the intervention.[22,23] This argument rests on the assumption that the intervention in question would benefit participants. However, as discussed above, not all sexual health promotion interventions (or interventions tested in RCTs) are effective, and some may cause significant harm. When a state of equipoise exists, that is, when there is uncertainty about whether potential trial participants would benefit or be harmed by being in one arm of a proposed trial rather than another, it is ethical to undertake an RCT.[24] It has been argued that, in conditions of equipoise, randomization is *the most ethical* means of determining whether participants receive or do not receive an intervention of uncertain effectiveness and harmfulness. This is because RCTs are scientifically the strongest design and thus offer the best chance of reliably establishing whether or not interventions have particular effects.[25] The key issue is that, without the *controlled* experimentation of RCTs, the *uncontrolled* experimentation which is normal practice continues to prevail.[26] Several important ethical issues arise in trials of sexual health promotion. However, these issues also arise in clinical trials and do not render trials unethical. Where researchers seek to randomize individuals to different arms within trials, they must seek each participant's informed consent, both to be allocated in this way and to participate in data collection.[27,28] In the case of cluster trials (see Chapter 7) it is not feasible to seek individual informed consent to allocation, since communities rather than individuals are the unit of allocation. Individual informed consent to participate in data collection must still be sought in cluster trials. An additional ethical and scientific argument for RCTs is the use of randomization as a means of allocating inadequate levels of resources for a particular intervention, for example, with respect to the social intervention of day-care for preschool children in the UK.[29]

Where a certain standard of care exists, based on pertinent evidence that current care is appropriate and effective, participants in the control group of a trial of a new intervention should receive standard care, rather than no intervention.[30] This principle should apply equally to trials of health promotion and clinical interventions, and to trials conducted in developing and developed countries. In rare circumstances, cost or practical feasibility may mean that the current standard of care cannot be provided to participants in the control group. Where this is so, researchers must explain this to participants so that they can make an informed decision about whether they wish to participate in such a study.[27]

Epistemological arguments

Epistemology is concerned with the theory of knowledge. It has been suggested that experimental designs are inappropriate for investigating social activities,[31–33] including sexual health promotion,[34] because they embody a 'positivist' epistemology. According to Tones and Tilford (see Ref. 35, p. 52) 'positivism' involves a view of research that includes several key beliefs:

> the assumption that objective accounts of features of the world can be generated; the attempt to describe general patterns and elucidate … general laws; the proposal of unity of methods between the natural and social sciences; and the use of scientific method for the testing of hypothesis.

However, it is not at all clear that researchers can be slotted into a number of discrete epistemological frameworks, such as 'positivism'.[9] The notion that researchers fall neatly into frameworks that are incompatible with each other was made popular by Kuhn.[36] However, this view has been criticized by Bhaskar and others as too simplistic.[37] Hammersley[38] and Bryman[39] have both argued that social researchers do not fall neatly into 'positivist', or other, camps, but rather use a diversity of principles and methods that cannot be grouped into discrete frameworks.

Sexual health evaluators who advocate the use of RCTs might try to explore patterns of association between interventions and outcomes, that is, a positivist aim according to Tones' and Tilford's list above. However, these evaluators would not necessarily do so in order to develop general laws. Most experimental evaluators are likely to accept the contextual specificity of their findings and the need to collect and use process data to explore to where and when these findings *might* be applicable.[40] Few such evaluators would believe, as Kippax and Van den Ven[41] appear to suggest they do, that evaluations of interventions such as a condom promotion campaign aimed at Thai sex workers, or a negotiated safety campaign designed for Australian gay men, could provide globally generalizable evidence.

Similarly, experimental evaluations may not actually aim to produce an 'objective,' that is, investigator-centred, account of the world, as Tones,[32] as well as Featherstone and Latimer[33] have suggested. Researchers involved in experimental evaluations engage with participant-centred (i.e. 'subjective') accounts in a number of ways. Ideally, they develop their outcome measures on the basis of qualitative research, so that these have some meaning for researchers and participants alike, and conduct a process evaluation (see below) that examines the social practices involved in planning, implementing and living through an intervention.[9] Researchers can acknowledge that the meaning of sexual acts is socially constructed and will differ across contexts,[42] but are still able to explore some aspects of these acts (e.g. Did you wear a condom? Did you know your partner's HIV status?) using standard measures. Such measures may produce a pared-down sketch of a complex, socially constructed, and ever changing social world, but they are nonetheless useful. Thus, experimental designs are not inherently positivist.[42]

Another criticism, often linked to the critique of positivist epistemology, is that experimental designs assume too simplistic a view of causality. Nutbeam rightly suggests that health-related actions are 'caused' by a complex and constantly shifting range of factors, including but not restricted to, exposure to health promotion.[43] For example, whether a gay man has unsafe sex or not will be affected by a multitude of factors in addition to his exposure to sexual health promotion, not least the attitudes of his sexual partners.[44] Critics suggest that experimental evaluations attempt to ignore this complexity of causation.[41,43,45] The suggestion is that experimental evaluators set out to record whether individuals are exposed to an intervention or not, and then try to analyse whether this resulted in the hoped-for outcomes, while neglecting other, social influences on their actions and their health.[41]

However, this view is based on a total misunderstanding of experimental evaluation. Experimental designs are undertaken not to *ignore* all the other factors affecting participants, but to *take proper account* of them.[19] The very act of comparing an intervention group with a comparison group recognizes the complexity of causation of social action. It recognizes that social interventions work by interacting with the myriad other influential factors. In a sexual behaviour trial, for example, investigators assume that the practice of safer sex will be influenced by the type of sexual partner, and that the intervention and control groups should therefore, resemble each other in terms of their sexual partners. The aim is to see how the intervention *interacts with* and *contributes to* the broader picture, which includes sexual partners and everything else, rather than pretending that this picture does not exist. Experimental evaluations seek to examine the 'added value' that an interventions brings to sexual health outcomes across a population of individuals, rather than seeking to suggest that an intervention 'causes' a sexual health outcome in any one individual. Furthermore, far from being a recent import from biomedicine as anti-positivists sometimes suggest,[34] experimental designs have a long history in evaluating social interventions,[46,47] and their use in this field continues.[48]

Practical arguments

It has been suggested that allocation (random or otherwise) of participants to intervention and comparison groups is impossible in certain

circumstances: where there is user involvement or other community participation in the planning of the intervention;[4,41,43] interventions delivered via
community networks and structures;[31] and interventions addressing what
Caplan categorized as 'environmental' factors, and which others have termed
'structural' factors.[4,49,50] These difficulties have led some to conclude that
a preference for experimental designs often results in a concentration
on 'regressive' intervention methods.[51] The term 'regressive' here refers to
interventions that employ a single method which is developed without the
participation of affected individuals or communities, that is delivered in a
single institutional context and that addresses only the actions of individuals
rather than the wider social environment.

According to systematic reviews of sexual health promotion,[5,6] it does
indeed seem that the majority of rigorous experimental evaluations of sexual
health promotion has focused on simple and individual-based interventions.
However, these reviews also show that more complex community-based interventions have been evaluated using RCTs, and that many non-experimental
evaluations of sexual health promotion have also focused on interventions
that involved single methods and an individualistic approach.

There are examples of experimental or quasi-experimental evaluations of
'progressive' categories of intervention, that is, those involving user or community participation, those delivered via community networks, and those
addressing environmental/structural determinants of health. Concerning the
first category, Kegeles et al.[52] report an evaluation of an HIV prevention intervention that was developed collaboratively with users. In the second category,
Kelly et al.,[53] as well as Flowers and Hart[54] report on controlled evaluations of
sexual health promotion interventions delivered via peer education in community settings. Olsen and Farkas[55] and Hargreaves,[56] report completed or
ongoing evaluations of interventions that addressed environmental/structural
factors. Olsen and Farkas describe a matched controlled trial of the impact of
an employment creation programme on teenage pregnancy. Hargreaves
reports on an ongoing cluster RCT of a sexual health promotion intervention
aiming to improve South African women's socio-economic environment.
Village-based micro-credit schemes will be developed with the aim of enabling
impoverished women to develop increased economic independence, social
status, and power within sexual negotiations. There is thus no *necessary* relation between experimental evaluation and 'regressive' intervention; limited
imagination rather than experimental evaluation may be the main cause of
'regressive' interventions.

Others critics have argued that contamination between intervention and
control groups is a bigger problem for trials of sexual health promotion than

for clinical interventions.[41,57] In other words, there is more chance that control participants in sexual health promotion trials would be inadvertently exposed to the intervention under evaluation than would be the case in clinical trials. One approach to this potential problem is to allocate clusters or groups of people, rather than individuals, to intervention or control group (see Chapter 7). Examples of clusters used in experimental or quasi-experimental evaluations of sexual health promotion include: gyms;[58] schools;[59] and cities.[54] An intervention aimed at an intervention cluster could still affect a control cluster, for example, if residents in an intervention site travel to a comparison site and have sex or otherwise interact with its residents.[60] However, there is evidence that well-designed studies can avoid problems of contamination between intervention and comparison clusters by employing clusters whose residents do not intermingle,[54] or perhaps by statistically controlling for the effects of contamination.[61] It is also the case that cluster trials comparing randomized clusters run no greater risk of contamination than comparisons involving matched clusters.

These counter-arguments regarding allocation and contamination are not meant to suggest that allocation and contamination difficulties *never* impede or even prevent the use of experimental evaluations in the field of sexual health promotion. Instead, where these matters arise in a specific context, they should be the subject of empirically-informed assessment, which then informs a choice about research design, rather than topics for rhetoric attack and counter-attack.

Moving the debate forward

Considerable criticism has greeted the use of experimental evaluation of sexual health promotion.[9] It might be tempting for advocates of experimental evaluation to react by adopting a siege mentality and consequently ignore the value of using experimental methods alongside other evaluation methods, design trials without enough consideration of how many health promotion (compared with clinical) interventions aim to exert effects at both the individual and the community level, or forget that practical constraints may make experimental evaluation very difficult in the case of some interventions. However, a siege mentality and its consequent temptations should be avoided.

Experimental methods should be used alongside other evaluation methods because evaluations should not only aim to establish effectiveness. They should also explore *how* interventions work (or do not work) by undertaking integral process evaluations. Process evaluations should explore what needs (such as for knowledge or skills) the intervention is addressing, and how these are met. Process evaluations should also assess the facilitators and barriers to implementation and acceptance of the interventions. A recent example of the latter is a controlled trial of peer education for gay men in London, which had no apparent impact on HIV-risk behaviours.[58] Because the study had an integral process evaluation, the researchers were able to suggest possible explanations for intervention 'failure'; these centred on the unacceptability of the intervention to the peer educators who were asked to provide the intervention (see Chapter 13).

Process evidence should inform decisions about where, when and with whom an effective sexual health promotion intervention might be more generally deployed.[40] Process evaluation is not a 'bolt-on extra' (see Ref. 32, p. ii), but a necessary complement to outcome evaluation.

Sexual health promotion evaluators must not automatically opt for an individual-randomized trial of the sort generally (but not always*) used in clinical trials without first considering whether this is appropriate to the intervention in question. An individual's sexual health is determined by their social environment as well as by their own actions. For example, an individual's risk of HIV infection is determined not only by their own behaviour but also by the local prevalence of HIV, by the behaviour of their sexual contacts, and by the overall form of the networks within which they have sex.[62] Many sexual health promotion interventions aim to address both individuals and the social environments in which they exist. Individually-randomized trials are only of limited use in assessing the impact of such interventions because they examine only the effects of an intervention on an individual, not on a whole social environment.[63] The preferred design for experimentally evaluating sexual health promotion interventions of this sort is the cluster rather than individual randomized controlled trial.

Trialists must not forget the practical constraints on using experimental designs. As suggested earlier, the feasibility of using experimental designs to evaluate specific interventions should be the subject of empirically-informed assessment. As argued above, there is in principle no reason why most interventions cannot be subjected to experimental evaluation, even those that involve users or communities in planning, that work with community structures and that aim to bring about environmental or structural change. However, a minority of interventions will prove very difficult to evaluate experimentally. This often happens where it is politically unacceptable or

---

* Vaccine trials commonly used cluster designs since these also exert effects at an individual and population level.

practically impossible to deploy an intervention for some but not all of a population. It would have been highly problematic, for example, to evaluate the effect of lowering the age of consent for male homosexual intercourse by doing so in some areas of the UK, but not others. It would also be very difficult to undertake an experimental evaluation of the public health effects of sexual health promotion campaigns on national television, though some such studies have been undertaken.[9] Cluster trials may sometimes be impossible to undertake because a statistically adequate number of comparable clusters cannot be identified. A commitment to using experimental evidence should not lead to such 'difficult' interventions being ignored by researchers and policy-makers.[64] Where experimental evaluations genuinely are impossible, other methods, despite providing less clear evidence on effectiveness, *must* suffice.

Conclusion

Evaluating the effectiveness of sexual health promotion is necessary in order to promote the use of beneficial interventions, to prevent the deployment of harmful interventions, and to maximize the cost-effectiveness of programmes of sexual health promotion. Experimental methods are the most rigorous means of evaluating effectiveness, and should not be neglected because of dogma. Condemnations of experimental methods on grounds that they are positivist or encapsulate too crude a view of causality are themselves simplistic. The practical feasibility of undertaking experimental evaluation of sexual health promotion should be the subject of empirical assessment. Experimental evaluations of sexual health promotion should include process evaluations and allocation may often be of clusters rather than individuals. Sexual health promotion interventions that are not amenable to experimental evaluation, because of political or practical problems, should not be totally ignored by researchers and policy-makers. Where experimental designs cannot be used, other evaluation methods must suffice.

References

1. Hartley, M., Hickson, F., Warwick, I., Douglas, N., and Weatherburn P. (1999) *HIV Health Promotion Activity Map for Greater London 1999–2000*. Sigma Research/TCRU; London.
2. Caplan, R. (1993) The importance of social theory for health promotion: from discussion to reflexivity. *Health Prom Int*, **8**(2), 147–57.
3. Parish, R. (1995) Health promotion: rhetoric and reality. In: Bunton, R., Nettleton, S., and Burrows R. (eds) *The Sociology of Health Promotion*. Routledge, London, pp. 13–23.
4. Nutbeam, D. (1999) Oakley's case for using randomized controlled trials is misleading. *Br Med J*, **318**, 944–5.

5. Oakley, A., Fullerton, D., and Holland, J. (1995) Behavioural interventions for HIV/AIDS prevention. *AIDS*, **9**(5), 479–86.

6. Oakley, A., Fullerton, D., Holland, J., Arnold, S., France-Dawson, M., Kelley, P., and McGrellis, S. (1995) Sexual health interventions for young people: a methodological review. *Br Med J*, **310**, 158–62.

7. Christopher, F.S. and Roosa, M.W. (1990) An evaluation of adolescent pregnancy prevention program: is 'just say no' enough? *Family Relat*, **39**, 68–72.

8. Imrie, J., Stephenson, J., Cowan, F., *et al.* (2001) A cognitive behavioural intervention to reduce sexually transmitted infections among gay men: a randomized trial. *Br Med J*, **322**, 1451–6.

9. Oakley, A. (2000) *Experiments in Knowing: Gender & Method in the Social Sciences.* Polity, Cambridge.

10. Fitzpatrick, J. (1998) *AIDS Funding Research Bulletin 1: HIV Funding in England.* National AIDS Trust, London.

11. World Bank. (1997) *Confronting AIDS: Priorities in a Global Epidemic.* Oxford University Press, Oxford.

12. NHS Centre for Reviews & Dissemination. (1997) Preventing and reducing the adverse effects of unintended teenage pregnancies. *Eff Health Care*, **3**(1), 1–9.

13. Kleijnen, J., Gotzsche, P., Kunz, R.A., Oxman, A.D., and Chalmers, I. (1997) So, what's so special about randomization? In: Maynard, A. and Chalmers, I. (eds) *Non-random Reflections on Health Services Research.* BMJ Publishing Group, London, pp. 93–106.

14. Oakley, A. (1990) Who's afraid of the randomized controlled trial? In: Roberts, H. (ed.) *Women's Health Counts.* Routledge, London, pp. 167–94.

15. Stephenson, J.M. and Babiker, A. (2000) Overview of study design in clinical epidemiology. *Sex Transm Infect*, **76**(4), 244–7.

16. Guyatt, G.H., DiCenso, A., Farewell, V., Willan, A., and Griffith, L. (2000) Randomized trials versus observational studies in adolescent pregnancy prevention. *J Clin Epidemiol*, **53**, 167–74.

17. Deverell, K. (1995) KY Babies Peer Education Project Final Report. London: HIV Project, Camden & Islington Health Authority.

18. Kelly, J.A., St Lawrence, J.S., Betts, R.A., Brasfield, T.L., and Hood, H.V. (1990) A skills training group intervention model to assist persons in reducing risk behaviors for HIV infection. *AIDS Educ Prevent*, **2**, 24–35.

19. Stephenson, J. and Imrie, J. (1998) Why do we need randomized controlled trials to assess behavioural interventions? *Br Med J*, **316**, 611–13.

20. Des Jarlais, D., Goldberg, D., Tunving, K., Wodak, A., Hagan, H., and Friedman, S.R. (1993) Characteristics of prevented HIV epidemics. *IXth International Conference on AIDS/HIV STD World Congress*, Berlin, June 1993, Oral presentation, Abstract No. WS-C15–16.

21. Kelly, M. *Evidence into Practice: Challenges and Opportunities for UK Public Health Conference.* Health Development Agency & King's Fund, London, April 3, 2001, Chair's welcome.

22. Connell, D.B., Turner, R.R., and Mason, E.F. (1985) Summary of findings of the school health education evaluation. Health promotion effectiveness, implementation and costs. *J School Health*, **55**(8), 316–21.

23. Stimson, G.V. and Power, R. (1992) Assessing AIDS prevention for injecting drug users: some methodological consideration. *Br J Addict*, **87**, 455–65.

24. Wald, N. (1993) Ethical issues in randomized prevention trials. *Br Med J*, **306**, 563–5.

25. Chalmers, I. and Silverman, W.A. (1987) Professional and public double standards on clinical experimentation. *Control Clin Trials*, **8**, 388–91.

26. Chalmers, I. (1986) Minimizing harm and maximizing benefit during innovation in health care: controlled or uncontrolled experimentation? *Birth*, **13**(3), 155–64.

27. Bennett, R. (2001) HIV Research and informed consent: public health versus private lives. In: Doyal, L. (ed.) *Informed Consent in Medical Research.* BMJ Publishing, London, pp. 211–21.

28. Doyal, L. (1997) Informed consent in medical research: journals should not publish research to which patients have not given fully informed consent—with three exceptions. *Br Med J*, **314**, 1107.

29. Toroyan, T., Roberts, I., and Oakley, A. (2000) Randomization and resource allocation: a missed opportunity for evaluating health care and social interventions. *J Med Ethics*, **26**, 319–22.

30. Angell, M. (1997) The ethics of clinical research in the third world. *The N Eng J Med*, **337**, 847–9.

31. Downie, R.S., Tannahill, C., and Tannahill, A. (1996) *Health Promotion: Models and Values.* Oxford University Press, Oxford.

32. Tones, K. (1997) Beyond the randomized controlled trial: a case for 'judicial' review. *Health Educ Res*, **12**(2), i–iv.

33. Featherstone, K. and Latimer, J. (2001) Review of A. Oakley's experiments in knowing. Gender and method in the social sciences. *Sociol Health Illness*, **23**(6), 868–70.

34. Meyrick, J. and Swann, C. (1998) *An Overview of the Effectiveness of Interventions and Programmes Aimed at Reducing Unintended Conceptions in Young People.* Health Education Authority, London.

35. Tones, K. and Tilford, S. (1995) *Health Education Effectiveness, Efficiency and Equity.* Chapman and Hall, London.

36. Kuhn, T.S. (1970) *The Structure of Scientific Revolutions.* University of Chicago Press, Chicago.

37. Bhaskar, R. (1975) *A Realist Theory of Science.* Leeds Books, Leeds.

38. Hammersley, M. (1995) *The Politics of Social Research.* Sage, London.

39. Bryman, A. (1988) *Quantity and Quality in Social Research.* Routledge, London.

40. Peersman, G., Harden, A., and Oliver, S. (1988) Effectiveness of Health Promotion Interventions in the Workplace: A Review. Health Education Authority, London.

41. Kippax, S. and Van den Ven, P. (1998) An epidemic of orthodoxy? Design and methodology in the evaluation of the effectiveness of HIV health promotion. *Crit Public Health*, **8**(4), 371–86.

42. Bonell, C. (1998) Gay men: drowning (and swimming) by numbers. In: Hood, S., Mayall, B., and Oliver, S. (eds) *Critical Issues in Social Research: Power & Prejudice.* Open University Press, Buckingham.

43. Nutbeam, D. (1998) Evaluating health promotion—progress, problems and solutions. *Health Promot Int*, **13**(1), 27–44.

44. Davies, P. (1994) Acts sessions and individuals: a model for analysing sexual behaviour. In: Boulton, M. (ed.) *Challenge and Innovation: Methodological Advances in Social Research on HIV/AIDS.* Taylor & Francis, London, pp. 57–68.

45. Van den Ven, P. and Aggleton, P. (1999) What constitutes evidence in HIV/AIDS education? *Health Educ Res*, **14**(4), 461–71.

46. **Campbell, D.T.** (1998) *Methodology and Epistemology for Social Science. Selected Papers.* University of Chicago Press, Chicago IL.

47. **Boruch, R.F.** (1997) *Randomized Experiments for Planning and Evaluation: A Practical Guide.* Sage, Thousand Oaks CA.

48. **Petrosino, A., Boruch, R.F., Rounding, C., McDonald, S., and Chalmers, I.** (2000) The Campbell Collaboration Social, Psychological, Educational and Criminological Trials Register (C2-SPECTR). *Eval Res Educ,* **14**, 206–19.

49. **Aggleton, P.** (1999) *HIV at the Crossroads: Re-framing HIV Prevention.* National AIDS Trust, London.

50. **Parker, R.G., Easton, D., and Klein, C.H.** (2000) Structural barriers and facilitators in HIV prevention: a review of international literature, *AIDS,* **14**(suppl. 1), S22–S32.

51. **Nutbeam, D.** (2001) Assessing the effectiveness of public health interventions. *Evidence into Practice: Challenges and Opportunities for UK Public Health Conference.* Health Development Agency & King's Fund. London, 3 April, 2001, Oral presentation.

52. **Kegeles, S.M., Hays, R.B., and Coates, T.J.** (1996) The Mpowerment project: a community-level HIV prevention intervention for young gay men. *Am J Public Health,* **86**(8), 1129–36.

53. **Kelly, J.A.** (1997) Outcomes of a randomized controlled community-level HIV prevention intervention: effects on behaviour amongst at-risk gay me in small US cities. *Lancet,* **350**, 1500–05.

54. **Flowers, P. and Hart, G.** The gay men's task force: evidence-based sexual health promotion for gay men in the gay bars of Glasgow. *1st UK Health Promotion Research Conference.* Edinburgh, 6–8 April 1998, Oral presentation.

55. **Olsen, R.J. and Farkas, G.** (1991) Employment opportunity can decrease adolescent childbearing within the underclass. *Eval Program Plann,* **14**, 27–34.

56. **Hargreaves, J.** (2000) *Poverty & Development—An Approach to HIV Control in South Africa's Rural Northern Province.* Health Systems Development Unit, Acornhoek SA.

57. **Webb, D.** (1997) Measuring Effectiveness in Health Promotion. University of Southampton, Southampton.

58. **Elford, J., Bolding, G., and Sherr, L.** (2000) Peer education has no significant impact on HIV risk behaviours among gay men in London. *AIDS,* **15**(4), 535–8.

59. **Wight, D., Henderson, M., Raab, G., Abraham, C., Buston, K., Scott, S., and Hart, G.** (2000) Extent of regretted sexual intercourse among young teenagers in Scotland: a cross sectional survey. *Br Med J,* **320**, 1243–4.

60. **Bonell, C.** (1996) *Outcomes in HIV Prevention.* HIV Project, London.

61. **Torgerson, D.J.** (2001) Contamination in trials: is cluster randomization the answer? *Br Med J,* **322**(7282), 355–7.

62. **Anderson, R.M. and Garnett, G.P.** (2000) Mathematical models of the transmission and control of sexually transmitted diseases. *Sex Transm Dis,* **27**(10), 636–43.

63. **Hayes, R.** (2001) Can RCTs measure the endpoints in which we are interested? *Int J STD AIDS,* **12**(suppl. 2), 13.

64. **Davey Smith, G., Ebrahim, S., and Frankel, S.** (2001) How policy informs evidence: 'evidence-based' thinking can lead to debased policy making. *Br Med J,* **322**, 184–5.

Chapter 2

Sexual health interventions are unsuitable for experimental evaluation

Susan Kippax

Introduction

The argument advanced in this chapter is that most, if not all, sexual health interventions are inherently unsuitable for experimental evaluation. While it is possible to design interventions that can be randomized, in most cases the conditions demanded by experimental evaluation render either the interventions and/or the outcomes trivial. In particular, any behavioural change brought about by the intervention is likely to be transitory and/or insignificant. There may occasionally be significant outcomes, sometimes unintended, but these are, in general, exceptions. Furthermore, attempts to impose experimental evaluation distort both the evaluation process and, more importantly, the interventions themselves. It is argued here that assessment of interventions can be achieved, but by means other than experimental evaluation. Indeed, empirical evaluations of a descriptive kind are needed to evaluate the effectiveness of sexual health interventions.

Argument for unsuitability

Proponents of randomized controlled trials (RCTs), such as Oakley et al.,[1] and Aral and Peterman,[2] restrict the forms of acceptable evidence to such a degree that they commit researchers to adopting the equivalent of guidelines governing the evaluation of a drug or vaccine trial. My argument is that, in a number of very important ways, vaccines or drugs, or indeed any other physiological or physical intervention, are not the same as a sexual health intervention, that is, a non-clinical intervention that promotes sexual health. Researchers such as Speller et al.,[3] Tones,[4] Kippax and Van de Ven,[5] and Van de Ven and Aggleton,[6] have suggested a number of reasons why RCTs are unsuitable when applied to the evaluation of sexual health interventions.

Practical issues

Randomization and generalizability

Effectiveness is similar to, but different in important ways from, efficacy. While Aral and Peterman define effectiveness as '...the impact an intervention achieves in the real world, under resource constraints, in entire populations, or in specified subgroups of a population. It is the improvement in a health outcome...' (see Ref. 2, p. 33), they define efficacy as '...the improvement in health outcome achieved in a research setting, in expert hands, under ideal circumstances' (see Ref. 2, p. 33). In the case of sexual health promotion, random allocation of participants is so artificial a procedure that it results in an inability to generalize evidence that reports on the *efficacy* of an intervention amongst a study population, in order to guide decisions on *effective* sexual health promotion for 'normal' populations. The question of generalization from the laboratory to the field is left unexplored and unanswered by supporters of RCTs of sexual health promotion.

Isolating experimental and control groups

Furthermore, whether the context is the laboratory or the field, there are difficulties inherent in isolating the intervention and control groups from information and/or competing inputs from sources other than the message under evaluation. It is also difficult, if not impossible, to isolate the control from the intervention group, and to stop leakage from one to the other.

Cost and time concerns

Critics of sexual health RCTs, and others, such as Stephenson and Imrie,[7] point to the expensiveness of experimental manipulation and random allocation. A good illustration of the cost, in terms of funding and time, of experimental evaluation is the National Institute of Mental Health multi-site HIV prevention trial, entitled 'reducing HIV sexual risk behaviour'.[8] The study showed that a small group, seven-session HIV risk-reduction programme, which was between 90 and 120 min in length, conducted twice-weekly, and facilitated by people with previous experience of group-work who received extensive training, was effective.[8] Those receiving the intervention were more consistent condom users than those in the control group. However, the intervention and its evaluation took over one year, and involved a huge team of researchers and educators. While cost and time concerns do not make experimental evaluations inherently unsuitable (since not all sexual health interventions take place in a context of under-funding or of urgent pandemics, such as HIV), the generalizability and leakage issues noted above point to a more fundamental problem associated with experimental evaluation: relevance to the real world, another issue that Stephenson and Imrie raise (see Ref. 7, p. 611).

Conceptual issues

Focus on behaviour rather than social practice

People act with reference to meaning. They do not engage in sexual *behaviours* (e.g., penis-in-vagina), they enact sexual *practices* (e.g., they make love or have a one-night-stand). What distinguishes sexual practice from sexual behaviour is *meaning*. Meaning is not to be confused with cognition, in the sense of meaning residing in the mind of an individual (see Chapter 4). Meanings are essentially social, in that they are formed in the relations between people, a point to which I shall return in the next section.

While sexual behaviour may be reasonably similar across time and place, sexual practice differs. There are only a small number of sexual behaviours in which two or more people can engage: sexual intercourse (both vaginal and anal); oral–genital sex (fellatio and cunnilingus); and oral–anal sex; a number of more esoteric behaviours, such as sado-masochism; and a range of behaviours that involve touching/mutual masturbatory behaviours.

Sexual practice, on the other hand, is more fluid: it takes on a number of forms. Sexual practices are social and cultural practices, produced within particular historical times and places, and embedded in specific social formations.[9] Sexual practice is different in Australia than in France or Nigeria. It was different in medieval times than it is now. It changes depending on whether it is enacted within a stable relationship or a casual encounter; whether it is imposed, as in rape, or mutually agreed upon. It is different for men and women, and for heterosexuals and homosexuals. The meanings that inhere in sexual practice differ, not only across time and space, but also within a particular time and place in terms of the hegemonic, that is, dominant discourses. For example, the current discourses that frame sexual practice in the developed world are: the 'sex drive'; 'love and romance'; and 'permissive' discourses. The meanings of sexual risk differ in terms of how risk is understood and played out, with reference to the above sexual discourses and to discursive understandings of HIV and other sexually transmissible infections (STIs), and pregnancy.

Interventions aimed at changing so-called 'sexual risk' need to address the fluidity of meanings, they need to address sexual practice as it is lived. It is likely that HIV health promotion that simply addresses a behaviour, for example, condom use, misses the point, because it fails to take account of the varied social and cultural meanings of the practice. For example, the practice of condom use is different in the marriage bed from the practice of condom use in a brothel or a casual sexual encounter, although the behaviour is the same in all three contexts. Many public health approaches, which govern the ways in which interventions are developed and evaluations carried out, fail to take account of the meanings of sexual practice and sexual risk that are related, in a complex fashion, to the psycho-social and cultural realities of everyday life.

Furthermore, people act on health promotion messages and sexual health interventions in an active fashion. They are not patients; that is, they are not passive recipients of the intervention. When they act, their actions depend on the positions they take up with reference to the prevailing discourses of sex, love, and risk. Contemporary understandings of matters, such as HIV-transmission risk and viral load, influence the actions of some people, but not others. A person with HIV may act differently from someone who is HIV-negative, and a person who is HIV-positive, but with undetectable viral load, may act differently from someone with a high viral load. Recent evidence from ongoing research in Sydney indicates that many HIV-negative gay men rely on the insertive position when engaging in unprotected anal intercourse with casual partners whose HIV status they do not know.[10,11] One of the dilemmas facing those developing sexual health interventions targeting gay men is whether to acknowledge these sophisticated, but not necessarily safe, responses to current medical understandings of HIV-transmission risk and population viral load estimates.

The practices we are talking about are significant human practices, ones in which there is considerable psychological and emotional investment. This makes them difficult to change, unlike most commercial purchasing practices, where the advertiser is involved in the essentially frivolous task of persuading the buyer to choose brand X over brand Y. Sexual practice is extremely complex and its meanings dynamic, fluid, and changing.

As Chapman points out,[12] and Kippax and Van de Ven elaborate,[5] what all this means is that the requirement of experimental manipulation for an exact relationship between variables, that is, relating outcomes to trial arms, cannot be met. It can only be met if one assumes that sexual practice can be reduced to sexual behaviour, which it cannot. One cannot change sexual behaviour, because in the real world—outside the laboratory—there is no such thing. All sexual behaviour is sexual practice, that is, it is produced and enacted in particular interpersonal, social, historical, and cultural contexts.

Failure to treat individuals as social beings

Sexual health promotion interventions do not take place in a social vacuum: the people targeted are not individuals isolated one from the other, but social beings. Sexual practice typically occurs between two people, and the meanings of their practice must be negotiated and shared by each.[13] There is, however, another sense in which individuals are socially connected: the meanings that they negotiate are socially produced. So, although I accept, like Ramos and colleagues,[14] that health promotion should view sexual activity from the client's point of view, that is, address the client's meanings, it is very rarely the case that the client's meanings are peculiar to the client only, or indeed the client and his or her sexual partner. Focusing on a client's definition of reality, as endorsed by ethno-theory,[14] ignores the fact that an individual's sense of reality, or understanding of sexual activity, or conceptualization of risk, derive from their socio-cultural world. Meanings are constructed and elaborated in the exchanges between people located within their communities and societies. Interventions such as counselling, which focus on a single client, fall into the trap of methodological individualism. Such individualism treats persons as isolated from one another, and treats the social and cultural locations in which they act as factors that have to be controlled for in RCTs.

Persons are social beings.[15] Aiming at changing individuals makes little sense, as does distinguishing change at the individual, community, and societal levels. There is growing evidence that sustained individual change is not only part of, but dependent on, collective change, whether that be at the level of community or society. Sustained safer sexual practice is associated with supportive social norms and with community attachment.[16–18] If a person is a part of a collective, and a collective is made up of persons linked together in some way, culturally and socially, then interventions will, by definition, have potential influence at the individual, community, and societal levels. Such connectedness not only points the way forward for effective 'behaviour' change, but also provides yet another argument for claiming the inherent unsuitability of RCT evaluation. The so-called problem of 'leakage' or 'contamination' is, in fact, part and parcel of being.

This is why theories, such as the theory of reasoned action, discussed in Chapter 5, that assume a rational unitary human subject, and separate the intra-psychic from the interpersonal and social, fail to give an adequate account of sexual behaviour change.[19,20] It may also be the reason why voluntary counselling and testing interventions appear to be ineffective when targeted at HIV-negative persons, but appear effective with sero-discordant couples.[21] Counselling individuals to use condoms may strike a chord with sero-discordant couples, but such counselling is unlikely to be effective if the communities in which they live, work, and play, ignore or undermine such messages.

The accumulating evidence that change in sexual practice is aided and abetted by community activism, political will, and structural change, such as anti-discrimination laws,[22–24] also provides evidence for the inherent unsuitability of experimental manipulation. The difficulties of experimentally evaluating the effects of structural and environmental interventions are obvious. As Parker, Easton, and Klein, in their review of the literature on structural and environmental factors that affect HIV-prevention programmes,[25] point out: '...since by their very nature these interventions involve large-scale elements that cannot be easily controlled by experimental or quasi-experimental research designs' (see Ref. 25, p. S30).

Change can be produced in individuals, but usually by producing change in the collective at the same time. Indeed, to do otherwise makes the task at hand extremely difficult. There are some exceptions to this. One is in psychotherapy, although if this is to be effective, it generally takes a very long time. Another is in contexts where the person is isolated from his or her fellows. As Segal *et al.* have shown,[26–28] among repatriated US soldiers held prisoners-of-war, and Shallice has shown among Irish Republican prisoners,[29] change in important beliefs, values, and practices occurs when prisoners are isolated from their fellow prisoners. In these reports of persuasion and 'brain washing', there was systematic and persistent emphasis on the undermining of friendships, emotional bonds, and group activities, and information exchange was almost non-existent. These rather extreme examples illustrate the power of the social: social isolates are a comparatively easy target for behaviour modification and change, and the changes wrought are profound and long lasting.

What do these arguments mean for RCTs? Unless one can randomize communities and social groupings, both large and small, and at the same time address the dynamic and context-dependent nature of the meanings of sexual behaviour, RCTs and other experimental designs have no role at all in the evaluation of sexual health interventions.

The rise of the RCT in sexual health

Argument for 'rigorous' evaluations

In the light of these issues, why has there been a move to experimental evaluation, and why are RCTs regarded by many as the 'gold standard'?[30] The argument put by Oakley and others is that descriptive studies cannot answer questions about effectiveness.[30] RCTs '...provide a remedy to the inferential uncertainties of non-experimental designs' (see Ref. 31, p. 161). Furthermore, they note: '...RCTs are the most appropriate way of evaluating the effectiveness of behavioural interventions' (see Ref. 1, p. 484). Stephenson and Imrie likewise argue: '... randomization seeks to balance out external influences between groups so that the true effect of an applied intervention is detectable' (see Ref. 7, p. 612).

What RCT evidence shows

There have been a number of studies that employ experimental evaluation of the type considered appropriate by the above authors, that is, using the RCT design. Oakley et al.,[1] in their review of behavioural interventions for HIV/AIDS prevention, report that they located 68 separate studies, of which 18 were judged to be methodologically adequate. In another review, this time of sexual health interventions,[31] 12 of the 73 evaluations met their criteria of study design rigour. The major design problems identified by Oakley et al. were: use of non-equivalent control groups; failure to use randomized control groups; reliance on a pre- and post-test design; high attrition rates; and failure to discuss implications.[31]

Similarly, Jemmott and Jemmott,[32] who reviewed HIV sexual-risk behaviour intervention studies undertaken between 1990 and 2000, report 36 studies of behavioural interventions with heterosexual adolescents that included a control group and an assessment of HIV risk-associated behaviour. Only 23 of these studies used random assignment to experimental and control groups. They add that, in 13 of these, individuals were the unit of randomization, while, in 10, groups were the unit.

Stephenson et al., in their review of published trials that used, as the authors saw it, the most robust methodology for evaluating the effectiveness of behavioural interventions in HIV/STI prevention, could find only seven studies that met their criteria.[33] The criteria they used were: the intervention must be one designed to produce change in sexual behaviour; use of randomized allocation to intervention and control groups; and use of laboratory-diagnosed HIV/STI endpoints. They concluded that the disappointing results of the review reflected, at least in part '... the challenges involved in trialling complex interventions where causal pathways are not straightforward and the interventions themselves are often hard to develop and deliver as intended' (see Ref. 33, p. S122).

These reviews demonstrate that it is possible to carry out RCTs to evaluate the outcomes of sexual health interventions. However, a number of problematic issues are clear within these reviews. First, very few studies met the criteria of adequacy set out by the reviewers. Second, those that did almost invariably involved the random allocation of individuals or small groups of individuals to experimental and control groups. Third, the reviews report no conclusive evidence of the effectiveness of one type of intervention over another.

For example, the findings of the 12 research studies included in the Oakley *et al.* review,[31] indicate varying degrees of effectiveness of the interventions. Of those with a reasonably clear outcome, three were judged to have been effective, four partially effective, two ineffective, and one harmful. Similarly, of the seven studies judged to be methodologically sound in the review by Stephenson *et al.*,[33] only two of the seven showed clear evidence of effectiveness. One of these was one of the three interventions that involved one-to-one counselling, and the other was one of the four employing small group interventions. Jemmott and Jemmott are less succinct in their review,[32] but conclude merely that the interventions which focused on condom acquisition and usage were the most successful, while those advocating abstinence and reduction in numbers of sexual partners were the least effective. These findings are in line with previous reviews of non-experimental as well as experimental evaluations, such as that of Grunseit *et al.*,[34] which Jemott and Jemott fail to mention.

Oakley *et al.* conclude that inconclusive findings from the experimental studies that have been carried out simply point to the need for more research,[31] a strange request given the acknowledged difficulties inherent in the research. Kippax and Van de Ven suggest otherwise: 'An equally plausible interpretation ... is that the results of such studies are not generalizable: causes cannot be isolated and linked to particular outcomes or effects. Inferential certainty is not possible because of the complex nature of the communication/education process and the over-simplistic nature of the RCT...' (see Ref. 5, p. 376).

The practical problems discussed here illustrate the inherent unsuitability of RCTs. The paucity of RCTs does not simply '... reflect[s] the challenges involved in trialling complex interventions where causal pathways are not straightforward and where interventions themselves are often hard to develop and deliver as intended'. (see Ref. 33, p. S122). Rather, the conclusions of these reviews are illustrative of the issues raised in the last section. The experimental manipulations, if effective, remove the very stuffing, the social glue, that produces changes in beliefs, values and practices. Aral and Peterman talk of known confounding factors,[2] and Stephenson and Imrie of balancing out external influences between groups by using randomization.[7] These 'external influences' and 'confounding factors' are, however, the very things with which social scientist and educators must work. The focus of the interventions should be the interconnections between people, not individuals qua individuals. However, because experimental manipulation is difficult, most researchers and educators choose to randomize individuals or small groups, the latter usually being groups of isolates rather than socially constituted groups. One of the notable exceptions is Kelly *et al.* who reported the effectiveness of a peer-education intervention among gay men in community settings in some US cities.[35] Recent studies in the United Kingdom, using broadly similar methods, involving gyms in London, and cities in Scotland,[36,37] have failed to replicate these findings (see Chapter 13).

In general, then, the imposition of the experimental method leads to asocial interventions, both in the sense that behaviour rather than practice and, in general, the individual rather than the situated and connected person are targeted. The outcome of such targeting is, as has been shown, disappointing. There is a real risk that any changes brought about are superficial and short-lived. The social stuff, the stuff that makes people human, that identifies them as this or that sort of person, as heterosexual or homosexual, as male or female, as committed lover or casual sex partner, is omitted from the equation. People's locations and positions, the discourses that frame their understandings of their world, do contaminate and confound, but they lie at the very heart of what needs to be addressed. They should not be controlled or balanced out by experimental manipulation.

Problems of a different order

Category error

There is another problem with experimental manipulation: the application of an RCT to a sexual health, or indeed any behavioural, intervention involves, I believe, a category error in that there is a confusion about the 'message' and its 'adoption'.[38] In the case of a drug, efficacy can be evaluated under ideal conditions in the specific conditions of a trial, independently of the evaluation of effectiveness of use in the real world. However, a sexual health message cannot be evaluated independently of its adoption. In a very important sense, a message is not a message until it is read.

To illustrate my claim, consider the processes involved in evaluating, for example, the effectiveness of thick vs standard condoms, or of a particular drug treatment for HIV. I compare these with the processes of evaluating an intervention advocating sexual behaviour change. The question of whether thicker condoms are more effective than standard condoms should be, and indeed has been, tested by an RCT.[39] Volunteers are recruited, and individuals randomly assigned to the intervention and control arms. The outcome to be measured might be the number of condom breakages and/or the incidence of STIs in the two arms. The RCT aims to investigate whether thicker condoms are more or less effective than standard condoms, when adopted. The RCT does not aim to provide evidence about the uptake of condoms in the context of routine provision. Similarly for drugs, an RCT aims to determine the effectiveness of the drug, rather than uptake of the drug when routinely provided. With regard to uptake of either the thick condom or the HIV drug treatment, another study (a 'phase IV' study) would be undertaken to assess the likelihood of market take-up and popularity. RCTs are rarely, if ever, employed to do this.

In the case of a sexual health intervention, the separation of Phase III and IV (see Chapter 5) is, I believe, impossible. The message or intervention, say advocating condom use, cannot be evaluated independently of the message being adopted. In the trial of thick condoms, the mechanism, say comparative durability to friction, that makes thick condoms more, or less, effective than standard condoms, can be demonstrated independently of their adoption in the real world. However, the mechanism that makes for an effective or ineffective behaviour change message cannot be assessed independently of human agency and all that it entails, such as reflection and thought.

To equate the evidence-base of strategies, such as behavioural interventions or education advocating behaviour change, with drug effectiveness or the effectiveness of thick condoms, is to confuse the nature of evidence and to confuse paradigms. The latter interventions involve technical and material strategies, while the former involve the social and interpersonal strategies of human agents and their social and cultural understandings.

History

Historical change also acts to reduce the usefulness of evidence derived from RCTs of sexual health promotion. If thicker condoms are found to be more, or less, effective than standard condoms, then they will remain so over time, as well as in different populations. Similarly, the effectiveness of a drug is more or less independent of the historical time in which it is taken. It does not matter whether the drug is taken in 1938, 1988, or 2008. The same is not true of a behavioural intervention. A campaign advocating, for example, a message recommending 'a condom every time' has a different impact today than would a similar campaign had fifteen years ago. If a successful vaccine candidate were marketed tomorrow, the effect on the impact of such a campaign would be profound.

It is extremely difficult, if not impossible, to isolate the effects of an intervention from the overall ongoing changes occurring within particular populations arising as a result of other interventions, mass media messages, interpersonal communication, social mixing, and changes in the epidemiology of HIV and AIDS. What works now may not work in the next two or five or ten years' time. Many of the interventions deemed effective by Oakley *et al.* in their review of work would now be considered outdated and inappropriate.[31]

If the very same interventions are effective now but not tomorrow, if they work in Sydney's gay saunas, but not in London's gay gyms, then one wonders about the usefulness of experimental evaluation.

A way forward

Recognizing the inappropriateness of experimental methods

The various problems outlined above with regard to RCTs—category error, methodological individualism, and the absence of any appreciation of the socio-cultural or historical setting—loom large. My major claim is that these problems mean that the outcomes measured in RCTs of sexual health interventions are not, in principle, generalizable. It may be that the insistence on the part of some authors that experimental manipulation and RCTs are the 'gold standard' of evaluation is for no other reason than those making these claims know of no other methods, other than the clinical drug trial. Certainly, the language used by many of those who promote evidence-based health promotion and experimental evaluation has an uncanny resemblance to the language of the clinical drug trial. The term 'intervention' itself makes one think of a one-off event that either induces change or fails to do so, rather than a slow building of normative and cultural change. There is little room for the evaluation of entire programmes or national strategies that build over time, or of strategies that combine a number of interventions.

Health promotion is, however, something that builds over time, as for example, a serial cross-sectional study of the sexual practices of 17- to 19-year-old students at a university in Australia has illustrated.[40] This study showed that, although both the accuracy of students' knowledge and the safety of their sexual practice increased with time, from 1988 to 1994, and that there was no relationship between these two variables in any single year, there was a significant positive relationship between knowledge and practice over time. The findings are indicative of normative and cultural, but not individual, change.

The attempts by governments to combat HIV span years. National strategies are developed, and funding is committed for time periods of between five and ten years. Nation states can, and do, change laws and other rules regulating behaviour in order to ensure successful outcomes. Commenting on the range of interventions and harm reduction strategies,[24] Coates et al. (see Ref. 24, p. 1143) note that the:

> ...true impact was gained when they were applied simultaneously as part of community-wide efforts. A swift and effective community response depended on the pre-existing level of organisation in the community, the presence of gay

individuals in academia and public health, the ability of representatives of the community to achieve recognition and to establish links with the health system, and open-mindedness (in some countries) about homosexuality.

The pull of the clinic, and evidence-based medicine, is however very strong. Pointing to the need to base clinical practice on scientific evidence, Oakley *et al.* state that there is '... an equivalent need to base social interventions in health care, including health education and health promotion, on sound evidence' (see Ref. 31, p. 161). While I have no disagreement with this statement, Oakley and her colleagues go on to assert that the way to do this is to employ the RCT, so that the inferential uncertainties of non-experimental designs can be overcome. Taking up the language of the clinical trial, Jemmott and Jemmott use the term 'dose' when speaking of the duration of the intervention (page S43).[32] Similarly, Stephenson *et al.* seem to adopt the notion of a treatment naïve population group when they note that the baseline level of knowledge in the target population might influence the effectiveness of an intervention.[33] In particular, they entertain the notion that gay men who had been targeted by health promotion messages and interventions over the past decade or more might provide a greater challenge to evaluation, in the sense they mean it, than population groups that are relatively prevention naïve.[33] The language used by Aral and Peterman (see Ref. 2, p. 84) is instructive and, in their definition of effectiveness, there is an uncanny parallel with notions of uptake and compliance, as though the intervention was a treatment or a drug.

The adoption of the model of the clinical drug trial is inappropriate: the similarity between a drug and a sexual health promotion message is minimal. Not only is the adoption of the 'gold standard' inappropriate, its imposition brings with it a further problem, as Traynor observes.[41] In a very interesting and insightful paper, he draws a parallel between some styles of religious argument and the push for evidence-based medicine. The style, he says, involves a 'moral and intellectual discrediting of all those who do not join the promotion of its cause' (see Ref. 41, p. 155). Oakley and her colleagues equate the use of the RCT with methodological soundness.[31] In the same paper, they go on to argue (see Ref. 31, p. 161) that '[j]ournals should refuse to accept methodologically flawed papers' and '[f]unders should refuse to support studies with methodologically flawed designs'.[31]

Alternatives to experimental evaluation

Not accepting the RCT orthodoxy does not mean that evaluation and evidence-based practice is impossible to achieve in sexual health. One can evaluate the effectiveness of sexual health interventions by using methods other than RCTs. Programmes of interventions can be, and have been, evaluated using prospective, observational studies that rely on descriptive, rather than experimental, evidence.[2,6] Indeed, as I have argued, evaluations that take account of the particular and the local are far more likely to provide reliable assessments of the impact of health promotion and education.

The evaluation can take the form of building outcome indicators into ongoing research that monitors HIV disease and/or associated risk practice. Both cohort and cross-sectional studies have been used to evaluate the 'talk, test, test, trust' health promotion campaign. This campaign comprises one element of the 'negotiated safety' strategy embraced in Australia,[42,43] and the Netherlands,[44] in which unprotected sex between partners who are certain of their sero-concordancy, is promoted as one option for risk-reduction. Although such research cannot pinpoint the exact or particular health promotion message that was effective, it can provide a standard against which the ongoing health promotion programmes and strategies, national or local, can be evaluated. Similarly, the European cohort of sero-discordant heterosexual couples,[45] which showed that consistent condom use by HIV sero-discordant couples significantly reduced the risk of HIV transmission, is also providing evidence indicating the effectiveness of risk-reduction strategies.

The evaluation of whole programmes of sexual health education, rather than of comparatively short-lived interventions, takes time. Evidence is, however, slowly accumulating. In Australia, the evaluation of the National HIV/AIDS Strategy indicated that the strategic response has been effective.[46] On an international scale, after an examination of the evidence, the National Institutes of Health Consensus Development Conference concluded: '... [p]reventive interventions are effective for reducing behavioural risk for HIV/AIDS...' (see Ref. 47, p. S94). Reviews such as that by Grunseit *et al.* found that the accumulated evidence drawn from experimental, cohort, cross-sectional, and other descriptive studies, indicate the effectiveness of school education campaigns promoting safer sexual practices.[34] As Anderson has pointed out, we know that prevention works and we know how it works.[23]

Such descriptive approaches are extremely valuable in evaluating our successes and failures. Indeed there is every reason to use these inductive methods rather than make what I have argued are false assumptions about human behaviour and modes of changing it. Such non-experimental approaches not only give us some understanding of complex human practices, and ways of modifying them, but they avoid the pitfalls of constraining health education initiatives to those that can be experimentally evaluated. They also prevent researchers and evaluators deciding on the basis of an RCT that education does not work.

What are we to conclude, for example, from the recent experimental and quasi-experimental studies reported by Imrie *et al.*,[48] Elford *et al.*,[36] and Williamson *et al.*,[37] referred to above? None of these studies showed that the experimental arm of the study, the educational intervention, was effective, when compared with the control arm. Indeed the study by Imrie *et al.* showed that the intervention led to an increase, rather than a decrease, in the number of men presenting with STIs, although this effect attenuated over time.[48] Imrie *et al.* concluded (see Ref. 48, p. 1455–56) that:

> Despite its promise and acceptability, the brief cognitive intervention aimed at gay men at high risk of sexually transmitted infection did not reduce their risk of acquiring new infections. Even carefully formulated behavioural interventions should not be assumed to bring benefits. It is important to evaluate their effects in randomized trials using clinical end points wherever possible.[48]

We know that education does work: witness the extraordinary change in sexual practice of gay men in Australia, North America, and Europe. The evidence is there, as set out in a number of reviews.[23,24,49] The exact mechanisms are not clear-cut, but the careful analyses undertaken in these reviews identify the variables that are central to the changing of practice: the factors that promote and sustain, but not necessarily cause, change.

Conclusion

The orthodoxy of experimental manipulation and RCTs is dangerous when applied unthinkingly to health promotion. Like all orthodox positions, the present orthodoxy of the RCT has worked against effective health promotion, especially in the case of sexual health and other phenomena associated with complex human practices.

In the social arena, experimental manipulation is not useful and contains inherent weaknesses. Furthermore, the tools and conceptual frameworks being promoted by evidence-based medicine constrain what researchers and evaluators seek to know.[50] Use of these tools has meant that interventions are designed so as to make evaluation easy; a strategy that often leads to simplistic and sometimes trivial interventions. Those who insist on the superiority of experimental methods have unwittingly distorted health promotion efforts. While individuals, communities, and societies can change, and have changed, in their responses to sexual health promotion, interventions should not be aimed at any one of these levels. Interventions need to be aimed at the glue, the stuff that binds people and groups together. The focus should be the extant and living group or community. Interventions are most effective when they speak to people as they live their lives. Changes here will be more effective if supported by political acknowledgement and structural change.

Some authors, such as Clatts (see Ref. 51, p. 95) are pessimistic.[51] He writes:

> . . . that the process has gone terribly awry, that the undaunted search for quick-fix models forces us to crawl into very narrow boxes, that it jeopardises our ability to see the world as it is, as well as our ability to offer constructive ideas about how to change it. In my experience such models inevitably end up trying to fit the subject to the technology, rather than the other way around.

I think there is room for optimism. Health promotion can change, and indeed has changed, the way we all engage in sex. It has done this via a myriad of campaigns, messages, and medical advances, that are reported and mis-reported in the press and elsewhere. In the developed world, or at least in most of it, we have witnessed an unparalleled change in sexual practice, and risk of HIV-transmission has been reduced. We need to be able to show that this is the case and describe how we have managed it, not by applying models that do not fit, but by continuing to accumulate descriptive evidence. I am also optimistic that social scientists will continue to temper the excesses of their public health colleagues. I hope this chapter will open up the debate and go some way to moderate the orthodoxy.

References

1. Oakley, A., Fullerton, D., and Holland, J. (1995) Behavioural interventions for HIV/AIDS prevention. *AIDS*, **9**, 479–86.
2. Aral, S.O. and Peterman, T.A. (1999) Do we know the effectiveness of behavioural interventions? *Lancet*, **351**, 33–6.
3. Speller, V., Learmonth, A., and Harrison, D. (1997) The search for evidence of effective health promotion. *Br Med J*, **315**, 361–3.
4. Tones, K. (1997) Beyond the randomized controlled trial: a case for 'judicial' review. *Health Educ Res*, **12**, i–iv.
5. Kippax, S. and Van de Ven, P. (1998) An epidemic of orthodoxy? Design and methodology in the evaluation of the effectiveness of HIV health promotion. *Crit Public Health*, **8**, 371–86.
6. Van de Ven, P. and Aggleton, P. (1999) What constitutes evidence in HIV/AIDS education? *Health Educ Res*, **14**, 461–71.
7. Stephenson, J. and Imrie, J. (1998) Why do we need randomized controlled trials to assess behavioural interventions. *Br Med J*, **316**, 611–13.
8. The National Institute of Mental Health (NIMH) Multisite HIV Prevention Trial Group. (1998) The NIMH multisite HIV prevention trial: reducing HIV sexual risk behaviour. *Science*, **280**, 1889–94.
9. Haraway, D.J. (1991) *Simians, Cyborgs and Women: The Reinvention of Nature*. Free Association Books, London.

10. Rosengarten, M., Race, K., and Kippax, S. (2000) 'Touch wood, everything will be ok': Gay Men's Understanding of Clinical Markers in Sexual Practice. University of New South Wales/National Centre in HIV Social Research, Sydney.

11. Van de Ven, P., Kippax, S., Crawford, J., *et al.* (2002) In a minority of gay men, sexual risk practice indicates strategic positioning for perceived risk reduction rather than unbridled sex. *AIDS Care*, **14**, 471–80.

12. Chapman, S. (1993) Unravelling gossamer with boxing gloves: problems in explaining the decline in smoking. *Br Med J*, **307**, 429–32.

13. Ingham, R., Woodcock, A., and Stenner, K. (1991) Getting to know you... young people's knowledge of their partner at first intercourse. *J Community Appl Soc Psychol*, **1**, 117–32.

14. Ramos, R., Shain, R.N., and Johnson, L. (1995) 'Men I mess with don't have anything to do with AIDS': using ethno-theory to understand risk perception. *Midwestern Sociol Q*, **36**, 483–504.

15. Harre, R. (1979) *Social Being: A Theory for Psychology*. Basil Blackwell, Oxford.

16. Prieur, A. (1990) Norwegian gay men: reasons for continued practice of unsafe sex. *AIDS Educ Prev*, **2**, 109–15.

17. Kippax, S., Connell, R.W., Dowsett, G.W., and Crawford, J. (1993) Sustaining Safe Sex: Gay Communities Respond to AIDS. Falmer Press, London.

18. Tarr, C.M. and Aggleton, P. (1999) Young people and HIV in Cambodia: meanings, contexts and sexual cultures. AIDS Care, **11**, 375–84.

19. Kippax, S. and Crawford, J. (1993) Flaws in the theory of reasoned action. In: Terry, D.J., Gallois, C., and McCamish, M.M. (eds) *The Theory of Reasoned Action: Its Application to AIDS-Preventative Behaviour*. Pergamon Press, Oxford.

20. Ingham, R., Woodcock, A., and Stenner, K. (1992) The limitations of rational decision-making models as applied to young-people's sexual behaviour. In: Aggleton, P., Davies, P., and Hart, G. (eds) *AIDS: Rights, Risks and Reason*. The Falmer Press, London.

21. Weinhardt, L.S., Carey, M.P., Johnson, B.T., and Bickham, N.L. (1999) Effects of HIV counselling and testing on sexual risk behaviour: a meta-analytic review of published research, 1985–1997. *Am J Public Health*, **89**, 1397–405.

22. Auerbach, J.D. (1998) The role of behavioural research in HIV/AIDS prevention. *Curr Opin Infect Dis*, **11**, 3–7.

23. Anderson, R.M. (2000) Prevention Works. Plenary paper presented at the *XIIIth International AIDS Conference*. Durban, South Africa.

24. Coates, T.J., Aggleton, P., Gutzwiller, F., *et al.* (1996) HIV prevention in developed countries. *Lancet*, **348**, 1143–8.

25. Parker, R.G., Easton, D., and Klein, C.H. (2000) Structural barriers and facilitators in HIV prevention: a review of international literature. *AIDS*, **14** (suppl. 1), S22–S32.

26. Segal, H.A. (1954) Initial psychiatric findings of recently repatriated prisoners of war. *Am J Psychiatry*, **CXI**, 358–63.

27. Lifton, R.J. (1954) Home by ship: reaction patterns of American prisoners of war repatriated from North Korea. *Am J Psychiatry*, **CX**, 732–9.

28. Schein, E.H. (1958) The Chinese indoctrination program for prisoners of war: a study of attempted 'brainwashing'. In: Maccoby, E.E., Newcombe, T.M., and Hartley, E.L. (eds) *Readings in Social Psychology*. Methuen & Co., London.

29. Shallice, T. (1972) The Ulster depth interrogation techniques and their relation to sensory deprivation research. *Cognition*, **1**, 385–405.

30. Oakley, A. and Fullerton, D. (1996) The lamp-post of research: support or illumination? The case for and against randomized controlled trials. In: Oakley, A. and Roberts, H. (eds) *Evaluating Social Interventions*. Barnados, Ilford, Essex.

31. Oakley, A., Fullerton, D., Holland, J., *et al.* (1995) Sexual health education interventions for young people: a methodological review. *Br Med J*, **310**, 158–62.

32. Jemmott III, J.B. and Jemmott, L.S. (2000) HIV risk reduction behavioural interventions with heterosexual adolescents. *AIDS*, **14**(suppl. 2), S40–S52.

33. Stephenson, J.M., Imrie, J., and Sutton, S.R. (2000) Rigorous trials of sexual behaviour interventions in STD/HIV prevention: what can we learn from them? *AIDS*, **14** (suppl. 3), S115–S124.

34. Grunseit, A., Kippax, S., Aggleton, P., Baldo, M., and Slutkin, G. (1997) Sexuality education and young people's sexual behaviour: a review of studies. *J Adolesc Res*, **12**, 421–53.

35. Kelly, J.A., St Lawrence, J.S., Diaz, Y.E., *et al.* (1991) HIV risk behaviour reduction following intervention with key opinion leaders of population: an experimental analysis. *Am J Public Health*, **81**, 168–71.

36. Elford, J., Sherr, L., Bolding, G., Maguire, M., and Serle, F. (2000) Peer-led HIV prevention among gay men in London (the 4-gym project): intervention and evaluation. In: Watson, J. and Platt, S. (eds) *Researching Health Promotion*. Routledge, London.

37. Williamson, L.M., Hart, G.J., Flowers, P., *et al.* (2001) The gay men's task force: the impact of peer education on the sexual health behaviour of homosexual men in Glasgow. *Sex Transm Infect*, **77**, 427–32.

38. Ryle, G. (1949) *The Concept of Mind*. Hutchinson, London.

39. Golombok, S., Harding, R., and Sheldon, J. (2001) An evaluation of a thicker versus a standard condom with gay men. *AIDS*, **15**(2), 245–50.

40. Rodden, P., Crawford, J., Kippax, S., and French, J. (1996) Sexual practice and understanding of 'safe' sex: assessing change in 18–19 year old tertiary students. *Aust NZ J Public Health*, **20**, 643–8.

41. Traynor, M. (2000) Purity, conversion and the evidence based movements. *Health*, **4**, 139–58.

42. Kippax, S., Noble, J., Prestage, G., *et al.* (1997) Sexual negotiation in the 'AIDS era': negotiated safety revisited. *AIDS*, **11**, 191–7.

43. Crawford, J., Rodden, P., Kippax, S., and Van de Ven, P. (2001) Negotiated safety and other arrangements between men in relationships: risk practice redefined. *Int J STD AIDS*, **12**, 164–70.

44. Davidovich, U., de Wit, J.B.F., and Stroebe, W. (2000) Assessing sexual risk behaviour of young gay men in primary relationships: the incorporation of negotiated safety and negotiated safety compliance. *AIDS*, **14**, 701–6.

45. de Vincenzi, I. (1994) A longitudinal study of human immunodeficiency virus transmission by heterosexual partners. European Study Group on Heterosexual Transmission of HIV. *N Engl J Med*, **331**, 341–6.

46. Feachem, R.G.A. (1995) *Valuing the past… Investing in the Future: Evaluation of the National HIV/AIDS Strategy 1993–94 to 1995–96*. Australian Government Publishing Service, Canberra, Australia.

47. National Institutes of Health Consensus Development Conference Statement. Interventions to prevent HIV risk behaviours. *AIDS*, **14**(suppl. 2), S85–S96.

48. **Imrie, J., Stephenson, J.M., Cowan, F.M.,** *et al.* (2001) A cognitive behavioural intervention to reduce sexually transmitted infections among gay men: randomized trial. *Br Med J*, **322**, 1451–6.

49. **Rosenbrock, R., Dubois-Arber, F., Moers, M.,** *et al.* (2000) The normalization of AIDS in Western European countries. *Soc Sci Med*, **50**, 1607–29.

50. **Hopson, R.K., Lucas, K.J., and Peterson, J.A.** (2000) HIV/AIDS talk: implications for prevention intervention and education. *New Directions for Evaluation*, **86**, 29–41.

51. **Clatts, M.C.** (1994) All the king's horses and all the king's men: some personal reflections on ten years of AIDS ethnography. *Human Organisazation*, **53**, 93–5.

Chapter 3

The role of randomized controlled trials in assessing sexual health interventions

David A. Ross and Daniel Wight

Introduction

This chapter focuses on the role of randomized controlled trials (RCTs) of behavioural sexual health interventions in developing countries. It argues that, whenever feasible, well-conducted RCTs are the best method to evaluate the health and behavioural effects of such interventions. The appropriate use of designs such as cluster randomized trials makes it feasible to use experimental methods in the evaluation of a wide variety of sexual health interventions. However, we stress the fact that the dichotomy between advocates and detractors of experimental evaluation designs has often stemmed from both groups ignoring the simple fact that both RCTs and non-RCTs can provide useful and valid information. Blind rejection of one or other method is unhelpful; a poorly conducted experimental evaluation can give misleading results, conversely a well-conducted observational study can provide useful findings. Wherever possible we illustrate these arguments with examples from developing countries and explore the particular issues that affect evaluations in such countries. However, almost all the key arguments advanced here apply both in developed and developing country populations.

The advantages of RCTs

The key strength of any controlled evaluation is that secular trends, that is, changes over time in the outcomes of interest that are unrelated to the intervention being evaluated, are directly monitored within the control group. The inferences that can be drawn from such a study can be greatly strengthened by ensuring that other factors, known or thought to influence the outcomes of interest, are similar in both groups (intervention and control) before the intervention is introduced. However, even if the known and suspected variables are well matched across the arms of the trial, such quasi-experimental studies cannot take account of unknown factors that might influence the outcomes. This is the great strength of randomized controlled trials. If the allocation of the individual or group to the intervention or control arm is done randomly, this makes a controlled evaluation into a RCT. Provided the sample size and number of randomization units are sufficiently large, randomization will equalize the distribution of factors, known and unknown, that influence the outcomes of interest (see also Chapters 1 and 6). Random allocation is also one of the bases for the use of statistical significance tests of the differences observed between intervention and control groups.[1] Significance tests allow the assessment of the probability that observed differences between the intervention and control groups could have occurred by chance.

These advantages of RCTs over other evaluation designs, such as non-randomized controlled trials, before/after comparisons within the same individuals or groups, comparisons of outcomes in intervention adopters vs non-adopters, and case-control studies, are similar irrespective of the type of intervention being evaluated. However, there are two main reasons why the RCT is particularly appropriate for the evaluation of sexual behaviour interventions. First, there are considerable problems in measuring many individual, group and community factors that are thought to influence sexual behaviour (see Chapter 8). Survey data, which usually comprise the backbone of our information on sexual behaviour, are rarely validated, and cultural factors that may be important determinants of sexual behaviour are extremely difficult to quantify. Lack of knowledge about crucial determinants of sexual behaviour makes it very difficult to either equalize these potential confounding factors through matching at the start of the trial, or to take proper account of them in the analysis.

Second, there is little consensus on the mechanisms by which particular behavioural interventions may influence behaviour.[2] Information on factors that might influence sexual behaviour is especially scarce in developing countries because resources to carry out such research are so limited. The fact that such factors can be equalized by randomization is therefore especially advantageous in developing countries.

The RCT is, therefore, the evaluation design of choice for measuring the effectiveness of interventions. However, this does not mean that RCTs will always give valid or useful results. The validity of the findings from any evaluation design will not only depend on the design per se, but also on the quality and rigour with which it is implemented. The usefulness of the findings will depend very much on the suitability of the design to the particular intervention, the questions that the evaluation is attempting to answer, and the quality of both the intervention and its delivery. Other evaluation designs can and should contribute useful information about the potential of interventions.[3] They are essential in the development of programmes and their early, formative evaluation.[4] Once a particular intervention has been found to be effective, the focus of evaluation should change from evaluation of health and behavioural effects to evaluation of the coverage and quality of the intervention.[5] An example of this can be given from the field of vitamin A deficiency prevention programmes. Following a meta-analysis of eight trials of vitamin A supplementation, which showed a substantial impact on child mortality in developing country populations,[6] the focus of evaluation research rightly shifted to measuring whether programmes were achieving a high level of coverage of the target population with vitamin A supplements.[7]

Potential criticisms of RCTs of sexual behaviour interventions

The conclusion that the RCT is the evaluation design of choice for measuring the effectiveness of interventions is widely,[8–12] but not universally[13–16] (see Chapter 2) accepted. The major arguments advanced against RCTs are discussed below. Many of these issues also affect non-randomized or uncontrolled trials to an equal or greater degree.

Generalizing results from RCTs is impossible

The effectiveness of any intervention will be largely dependent on the specific context in which it is applied, irrespective of whether it has been allocated randomly or not. However, the collection of detailed baseline and process evaluation data from both intervention and control communities will help to explain this context and allow an assessment of the likely generalizability of both the intervention and the results to other populations. Such detailed information is, of course, equally important whether or not the intervention has been randomized.

Whenever possible, more than one well-conducted experimental evaluation should be undertaken to test the degree to which the results can be generalized across locations and cultures. Careful examination of the potential reasons for any differences found (e.g. in the characteristics of the populations, the interventions or outcomes etc.) helps to clarify the necessary conditions for the intervention to be effective. For example, two recent RCTs of the introduction of treatment of sexually transmitted infections (STIs) in East Africa produced very different results.[17,18] In a trial in Mwanza Region of Tanzania, the introduction of improved STI case management using the syndromic management approach in rural government clinics reduced the incidence of HIV in adults in the surrounding communities by 38 per cent (95% CI −15, −55%) relative to control communities.[17] Conversely, in an RCT in Rakai District in neighbouring Uganda, the introduction of directly-observed mass treatment of all adults every 10 months with highly effective, single dose oral antibiotics and treatment of all individuals who tested positive for syphilis resulted in only a non-significant 3 per cent lower (95% CI −16,+19%) incidence of HIV in the intervention communities.[18] The reasons for these contrasting findings have been the subject of intense debate that has led to important new hypotheses about the mechanisms of the STI cofactor effect in the transmission of HIV.[19]

Large-scale studies obscure the distinct needs of different subgroups

It is sometimes argued that experimental evaluations of behavioural interventions rarely demonstrate a positive effect because the intervention group is too heterogeneous. The argument is that the intervention might work with specific sections of the target population, but the need for a large sample means that the positive effect on some is obscured by no effect or a negative effect on others. This can be a serious criticism in an affluent country where it might be possible to target specifically tailored interventions for different sub-groups. Clearly, if such a situation is expected, one should try to make separate evaluations of specifically-targeted interventions, rather than a blunderbuss evaluation of a single intervention administered to varied sub-groups, some of whom are thought unlikely to benefit from it. This is the case, irrespective of the evaluation design. Alternatively, sub-group analysis can be performed to investigate the impact of the intervention within specific sub-groups, especially where these have been decided in advance and are based on a priori hypotheses and a sufficiently large sample. In practice, this is a relatively rare concern in the developing world where the scale of sexual health problems is so great, and resources so scarce, that mass interventions (e.g. standardized school sex education), are often the only feasible strategy.

Random allocation is unavoidably, and wastefully, expensive

Random allocation does not necessarily increase the cost of a trial, especially when cluster randomization is used. Usually, the major costs stem from the direct costs of the intervention and its development, and the assessment of outcomes, especially if these include laboratory tests for biological outcomes. When outcome evaluations are deemed necessary, it is extremely wasteful to go to this expense without adopting, if possible, a randomized design, which greatly increases the validity of the findings. If it is argued that the expense of outcome evaluations is not justified, then this cost must be compared with that of continuing potentially ineffective or even harmful programmes indefinitely.

It is difficult to isolate the intervention group from other information or inputs

Totally isolating the intervention group from other sexual health information or inputs is usually impossible in any evaluation of an intervention. However, this is particularly problematic for uncontrolled and non-randomized trials. Within an RCT that has an adequate number of randomization units, external or pre-existing influences will, on average, affect the intervention and control groups equally, whether or not they have been measured. Other influences or inputs are therefore much less of a problem for RCTs than for non-randomized trials. Furthermore, the detailed process evaluation that should be a component of any intervention evaluation should measure those external influences.

It is impossible to stop the intervention leaking into the control group

Leakage or spill-over of the intervention into the control group will reduce the chances of finding a true, causal difference between the two groups. However, once again, the risk of such contamination is not peculiar to RCTs, but needs to be considered in any controlled evaluation. Spill over is not inevitable and can be avoided or minimized by the selection of appropriate trial communities. For example, investigators in the MEMA kwa Vijana trial in Tanzania ensured that there were 'buffer' communities which did not receive the new intervention between the communities selected for randomization to intervention or control groups (see Chapter 11).[20] In developing countries, where the mass media and transport infrastructure are usually less well developed, the risks of spill-over are often less serious than in developed countries. Nevertheless, the possibility of contamination makes it more difficult to evaluate the impact of programmes that include the use of mass media approaches.

Random allocation reduces the degree of benefit that comes from an individual or group actively choosing to participate in the particular intervention

Willingness to participate in a particular intervention can have a substantial impact on its effects, and so self-selection into intervention groups gives quasi-experimental studies a greater chance of positive results.[21] However, when the aim of the evaluation is to measure the effectiveness of an intervention among all potentially eligible individuals, 'randomizing out' the self-selection effect can be seen as an advantage. Even when self-selection is an intrinsic part of the intervention (e.g. a couple choosing between the use of female or male condoms), sophisticated research designs may still be able to combine an element of choice within a randomized design (see Chapter 6). For example, male and female condoms could be offered to all the couples who could then choose to try neither, one or other or both (each option lasting, say, for 6 months). Those choosing either the male or the female condom would receive that intervention. Those willing to try both types of condom would then be randomly allocated to either receive the male or the female condom first. Outcomes such as client satisfaction and contraceptive failure or STI rates in those using the male versus the female condom could be compared in each of the two trial periods. Other useful information could be gained by comparing outcomes between those who only chose one type of condom and those who chose neither. The latter would be a non-randomized trial, and the results would need to be interpreted with that in mind.

The quality of the intervention is often assumed, simply because it has been the subject of an RCT

The quality of the intervention and the quality of its evaluation must never be assumed, irrespective of the evaluation design. Detailed quality assessments should be made both before and during the intervention evaluation period. It is also important to investigate which components of the intervention appear to have been more effective than others, through detailed process evaluation (see Chapter 10).

A further possible problem is that a potentially effective, high quality intervention may not have actually been delivered to, or taken up by, the intended beneficiaries. The degree to which this has occurred can usually be measured during the trial. The main analysis of the trial results should be based on a comparison of outcomes in all the individuals (or groups of individuals) who were randomly allocated to receive the intervention vs those who were randomly allocated to be in the control group (i.e. an intention to treat analysis). This gives a measure of the effectiveness of the intervention in the whole group of people who could have received it, irrespective of whether they actually did. Other useful information can be gained by looking at the impact among those who actually received or participated in the intervention. Care needs to be taken, however, when interpreting such 'on-treatment' or 'participants only' results, especially if there is no equivalent participants only group within the control arm. Compliers usually have much more favourable outcomes than non-compliers, even if the intervention they complied with is totally ineffective. In a drug trial, it is easy to ensure that there is an equivalent group of compliers within the control group. Outcomes in those individuals who took all the expected doses of the test drug can be directly compared with those who took all the expected doses of the comparison treatment or a placebo. In some sexual behaviour intervention trials, a similar comparison is also possible. For example, in a trial comparing a new sex education curriculum with an existing curriculum, an on-treatment analysis could compare participants who attended at least 90 per cent of the sessions of the new curriculum vs those who attended at least 90 per cent of the comparison curriculum. However, where the comparison is with no sex education at all, such an on-treatment analysis would necessarily lose the balance between the intervention and control arms, as there would be no equivalent group of compliers within the control arm. Although the outcome results could be adjusted for independent variables that predict the main outcomes in a multivariate analysis, biases might remain because of differences between the two arms in unknown confounders or in variables that were not measured.

Prioritizing evidence from experimental designs belittles the value of interventions that cannot be randomized

If policy makers accept that the best evidence of effectiveness comes from carefully designed experimental evaluations then there is a danger they might attach little importance to the outcomes from non-experimental evaluations. Some programmes are not well-suited to randomized trials, such as mass media programmes or those initiated by lay community groups, yet it is theoretically possible that these might be the most effective. Policy makers should not, therefore, let their choice of interventions be determined entirely by the rigour of evaluation design. It is a very important factor in the weight of evidence for or against the effectiveness of an intervention, but not the sole factor.

It is ethically unacceptable to deny the intervention to the control arm in a trial

A further argument that has been made against randomized controlled trials is that it is often unethical to withhold the intervention from the control group (see Chapter 1). In as much as it is valid, this criticism applies to any form of prospective evaluation that includes a control group. This argument only holds if there is strong, pre-existing evidence that the intervention has positive benefit. Within the field of sexual behaviour interventions, this is rarely the case. For example, the evidence that any specific sexual behaviour intervention in developing countries has had a beneficial impact among adolescents is conspicuous by its absence.[22]

Conversely, the possibility that interventions could have negative effects should not be summarily dismissed. For example, a frequently heard criticism of adolescent sex education is that legitimizing the discussion of sex and sexuality could lead to adolescents experimenting more with sex. Similarly, it has been argued that providing clear information that contraceptives can reduce the risk of pregnancy might remove a major barrier to adolescents having sex. In sub-Saharan Africa, another widely held view is that sex education might give teachers more opportunity to sexually exploit their students, a practice that has been widely documented.[23,24] More generally, it is salutary to note that in several different fields social interventions that were widely assumed to be beneficial have been found to have damaging effects.[12]

In a situation where there is no clear evidence as to whether the intervention will have beneficial, neutral or harmful effects, a RCT is both ethical and needed. The limited empirical data that can be brought to bear on these arguments come almost entirely from research in developed countries.[22] Furthermore, most developing countries have few pre-existing sexual behaviour interventions in place and limited resources available to introduce such interventions. Therefore, it is rarely the case that an RCT requires withholding from people an intervention that they would otherwise have received.

RCTs do not last long enough to demonstrate effectiveness

Achieving a measurable impact within the usual time frame of most intervention evaluations is difficult. Hence, it is possible that a lack of measured impact within the evaluation period may not reflect a true impact that would take longer to achieve. Long-term follow-up should be carried out whenever possible, but effective interventions to reduce HIV, STIs and unwanted pregnancies are needed urgently, especially in many developing countries. For example, the HIV epidemic is progressing so rapidly in many countries, and the burden from other reproductive health problems is so great, that it can reasonably be argued that priority needs to be given to interventions that will have a substantial beneficial impact within five to ten years.

Randomization is not always feasible

There are three main types of interventions that are usually unsuitable for evaluation within an RCT. First, some interventions cannot be restricted to a circumscribed intervention group, such as mass media programmes. Second, the mechanism by which some interventions are supposed to work involves the programme's initiation by the target group themselves. If it were to be prescribed from above, which would be necessary in a randomized trial, it would exclude an essential element of the programme. Third, some target groups, such as street children or lorry drivers, can be highly mobile. Longitudinal studies of any sort that involve repeated contacts with the same individuals over a prolonged period may fail due to excessive attrition or loss during follow-up.

RCTs require standardized programmes

A further difficulty with large-scale evaluations, whether experimental or not, is that ideally they evaluate a standardized programme so it is clear what, exactly, the intervention has been. However, many practitioners would argue that behavioural programmes must be adapted for the particular experiences and maturity of the groups with which they work. Once again, this issue affects both non-randomized and uncontrolled evaluations as much as RCTs. Clearly, the overall result will be an evaluation of the overall intervention, and interpretation of the results will need to take account of any modifications during the evaluation period. If these have been substantial, the results among subgroups that received the original and the modified intervention should be compared. The content and techniques used in the intervention, including any modifications during the trial, should be documented in detail. This should be reported so that others can also assess the actual intervention that has been evaluated.

Other issues concerning the role of randomized trials of sexual health interventions

Exploratory research and the timing of RCTs

Before considering a trial, a detailed review of evidence relating to the appropriateness and effectiveness of the intervention should be conducted. If no research has been conducted on its likely effectiveness then preliminary assessments of this should be made. Appropriateness should acknowledge realistic restrictions on cost, so that it could be replicated and sustained. Such developmental research is necessary to ensure that the most promising intervention is subjected to a trial. RCTs are not appropriate for exploratory research into these factors.[11] Qualitative and quantitative observational studies are necessary to clarify the mechanisms by which the intervention is meant to work, the contexts necessary for this to happen, and how the target group might respond to it. These points are discussed in greater detail in Chapters 4 and 5.

It should be recognized that our knowledge in this field is incremental, and it is a myth to think that one would ever reach the stage where one fully understands which kind of intervention is likely to be the most effective. Where there are clear gaps in our knowledge, a balance will need to be struck between the desire for further preliminary research and the delay this will cause to the start of the trial, and hence to the introduction of the intervention. The gravity of sexual health problems in developing countries may lead researchers and practitioners to initiate trials at an earlier stage than they might do in countries with much lower morbidity and mortality (see Chapter 11).

Imperfect validity and potential biases in outcome measures

All evaluations of sexual behaviour interventions, whether observational or experimental, must overcome the problems inherent in the measurement of outcomes, including imperfect validity of most behavioural, clinical, and biological outcome indicators (see Chapters 8 and 9). However, to some extent, randomization again reduces this problem. Providing the trial is large enough, randomization should ensure equal distribution of most biases, including the imperfect validity of outcome measures, between the intervention and control groups. One advantage for evaluators in developing countries is that the biological and clinical outcomes of interest are often, tragically, much more common (e.g. HIV/AIDS and other STIs, unwanted pregnancy). This makes it much more feasible to include such relatively 'hard' outcomes in these contexts.

Evaluation of multi-component interventions

In many situations, single interventions may not be sufficient to achieve a substantial change in sexual behaviour. But multi-component intervention packages, for example, a combination of health service initiatives, face-to-face health education in schools and in the community, plus mass media health education, are complex to implement and are likely to be expensive. They are much more complex than specific medical treatments, often needing group, institutional or societal change as well as individual changes in attitudes and behaviour. Often, it will be difficult to separate the impact of the various components of the intervention package. This argues for a detailed evaluation of all the major processes that would need to occur for the intervention to have an effect. This detailed process evaluation is essential to interpret the main results of the trial and is discussed in more detail in Chapter 10. For example, an intervention trial might include a component of classroom-based sexual and reproductive health education by teachers and the main outcomes of the trial could be the frequency of HIV, other STIs, and unwanted pregnancy in participants. In addition to the main behavioural, clinical and biological outcomes, such a trial should also include an evaluation of the:

- quality of the materials used to train the teachers
- quality of the materials used by the teachers
- quality of the training of the teachers
- quality of the teaching itself
- number and proportion of sessions taught
- perceptions of the participants related to these sessions
- impact of the teaching on the knowledge, attitudes and reported behaviours of the participants.

This process evaluation should help to assess which of the sessions or key messages have been effective and which have not.

What are the hallmarks of a good RCT?

The trial evaluates a high-quality intervention

There is little point in introducing a low-quality intervention, and even less point in setting up an RCT to evaluate such an intervention. A trial should only be initiated when the supposed mechanism and necessary context for the intervention have been clearly articulated, and there is good research evidence that it may be effective. However, the resources available to maintain the intervention in the trial communities after the evaluation, let alone to replicate it on a large scale, may be very limited in developing countries. The trial intervention should therefore be designed with this in mind. Should the intervention be effective, it should be possible to apply these results within programmes outside the trial setting (see Chapter 12).

The trial answers important, relevant questions and uses an ethical control group

An RCT should be designed to answer an important and relevant question. It is usually a waste of time and resources to evaluate an intervention that could never be implemented on a large-scale with individuals or communities similar to those who participate in the evaluation. The heated debate over whether control groups in developing countries should receive the same standard of care as they would receive in developed countries is less pressing within the field of behavioural intervention research than in clinical intervention trials.[25–29] This is because the evidence that any sexual behavioural interventions have worked is weak, let alone that they have worked within the particular social and cultural contexts of specific developing countries.

Given that such contexts are so important to the likely effectiveness of sexual behaviour interventions, the contexts assume much greater significance than for trials of drugs.

The trial measures outcomes with proven high validity

Measuring outcomes with low validity will give misleading results, whatever the design of the study. Furthermore, the blind use in developing countries of outcomes and measurement methods that have only been validated in developed countries may give misleading results. For example, the validity of answers from self-completion questionnaires will be at least partially dependent on levels of literacy and the understanding of the concepts and terminology; the acceptability of taking biological specimens needs to be established in the specific population under study; and the use of telephone or postal questionnaires may not be an option, particularly in developing country settings (see Chapter 8). Given the problematic nature of measuring sexual behaviour, it will be advisable to include biological, and possibly, clinical outcome measures as well as behavioural ones, even if this increases the cost substantially. The relatively high prevalence and incidence of such outcomes in most developing countries often makes this feasible, if expensive.

The trial has adequate sample size and power

Careful consideration needs to be given to ensuring that the sample size is adequate for the trial to be able to detect a true impact on outcomes of public health importance. With many developing country populations, such trials have two major design advantages over equivalent trials in developed countries—the scale of sexual and reproductive health problems is often orders of magnitude greater, and, conversely, the quality and intensity of existing interventions is often woefully inadequate or non-existent. This makes the chances of a new intervention having a substantial and measurable effect much greater. Particular consideration of sample size is needed for cluster randomized trials (see Chapter 7).

The trial includes adequate evaluation of the intervention and its delivery

Published reports of evaluation results rarely give sufficient detail of the actual intervention to be able to judge its quality and coverage. However, it is usually possible to document this within other publications, to give further details in electronic format on a journal's web page, and to make the intervention materials, the results of internal and external process evaluations, and data on the coverage of the intervention available to readers on application.

External factors that could influence the trial outcomes are carefully documented in both groups

This will usually require specific data collection within both intervention and control communities before and during the trial.

The trial uses culturally sensitive intervention and evaluation designs

Both the intervention and evaluation design must be tailored to the cultural setting in which the trial is taking place.

Conclusions

RCTs are the preferred method for the evaluation of the behavioural and health effects of behavioural sexual health interventions. Furthermore, appropriate use of designs such as cluster randomization make it feasible to use the RCT design in the evaluation of many, possibly most, sexual behaviour interventions.

References

1. Brennan, P. and Croft, P. (1994) Interpreting the results of observational research: chance is not such a fine thing. *Br Med J*, **309**, 727–30.
2. Turner, G. and Shepherd, J. (1999) A method in search of a theory: peer education and health promotion. *Health Educ Res*, **14**, 235–47.
3. Kirkwood, B.R., Cousens, S.N., Victora, C.G., and de Zoysa, I. (1997) Issues in the design and interpretation of studies to evaluate the impact of community-based interventions. *Trop Med Int Health*, **2**, 1022–9.
4. Davies, H., Nutley, S., and Tilley, N. (2000) Debates on the role of experimentation. In: Davies, H., Nutley, S., and Smith, P. (eds) *What Works?* Policy Press, Bristol UK.
5. Habicht, J.P., Victora, C.G., and Vaughan, J.P. (1999) Evaluation designs for adequacy, plausibility and probability of public health programme performance and impact. *Int J Epidemiol*, **28**, 10–18.
6. Beaton, G.H., Martorell, R., L'Abbe, K.A., Edmonston, B., McCabe, G., Ross, A.C., and Harvey, B. (1993) *Effectiveness of Vitamin A Supplementation in the Control of Young Child Morbidity and Mortality in Developing Countries*. United Nations, ACC/SCN Nutrition Policy Discussion Paper No. 13, Geneva.
7. Ross, D.A. (1998) Vitamin A and public health: challenges for the next decade. *Proc Nutr Soc*, **57**, 1–8.
8. Oakley, A. and Fullerton, D. (1996) The lamp-post of research: support or illumination? The case for and against randomised controlled trials. In: Oakley, A. and Roberts, H. (eds) *Evaluating Social Interventions*, Barnados, Ilford, Essex.
9. Green, S.B. (1997) The advantages of community-randomized trials for evaluating lifestyle modification. *Control Clin Trials*, **18**, 506–13.
10. Rothman, K.J. and Greenland, S. (1997) *Modern Epidemiology*. Lippincott-Raven, Hagerstown, USA.

11. **Stephenson, J. and Imrie, J.** (1998) Why do we need randomised controlled trials to assess behavioural interventions. *Br Med J*, **316**, 611–13.

12. **MacIntyre, S. and Petticrew, M.** (2000) Good intentions and received wisdom are not enough. *J Epidemiol Commun Health*, **54**, 802–3.

13. **Pawson, R. and Tilley, N.** (1997) *Realistic Evaluation.* Sage, London.

14. **Speller, V., Learmonth, A., and Harrison, D.** (1997) The search for evidence of effective health promotion. *Br Med J*, **315**, 361–3.

15. **Tones, K.** (1997) Beyond the randomised controlled trial: a case for 'judicial' review. *Health Educ Res*, **12**, i–iv.

16. **Kippax, S. and Van de Ven, P.** (1998) An epidemic of orthodoxy? Design and methodology in the evaluation of the effectiveness of HIV health promotion. *Crit Public Health*, **8**, 371–86.

17. **Grosskurth, H., Mosha, F., Todd, J.,** *et al.* (1995) Impact of improved treatment of sexually transmitted diseases on HIV infection in rural Tanzania: randomised controlled trial. *Lancet*, **346**, 530–6.

18. **Wawer, M.J., Sewankambo, N.K., Serwadda, D.,** *et al.* (1999) Control of sexually transmitted diseases for AIDS prevention in Uganda: a randomised community trial. *Lancet*, **353**, 525–35.

19. **Grosskurth, H., Gray, R., Hayes, R.,** *et al.* (2000) Control of sexually transmitted diseases for HIV-1 prevention: understanding the implications of the Mwanza and Rakai trials. *Lancet*, **355** (World AIDS Supplement), WA8–WA14.

20. **Ross, D.A., Obasi, A., Changalucha, J.,** *et al.* Community-randomized trial of an intervention to prevent HIV infection and enhance reproductive health among adolescents in rural Tanzania. *XI International Conference on AIDS and STDs in Africa.* Lusaka, Zambia, 12–16 September 1999, Abstract 15PT15-15.

21. **Guyatt, G.H., DiCenso, A., Farewell, V., Willan, A., and Griffith, L.** (2000) Randomized trials versus observational studies in adolescent pregnancy prevention. *J Clin Epidemiol*, **53**, 167–74.

22. **Grunseit, A.** (1997) *Impact of HIV and Sexual Health Education on the Behaviour of Young People: A Review Update.* UNAIDS, Geneva.

23. **Kuleana.** (1999) *The State of Education in Tanzania: Crisis and Opportunity.* Kuleana Centre for Children's Rights, Mwanza, Tanzania.

24. **Shumba, A.** (2001) Who guards the guards in schools? A study of reported cases of child abuse by teachers in Zimbabwean secondary schools. *Sex Educ*, **1**, 77–86.

25. **Lurie, P. and Wolfe, S.M.** (1997) Unethical trials of interventions to reduce perinatal transmission of the human immunodeficiency virus in developing countries. *N Engl J Med*, **337**, 853–6.

26. **Angell, M.** (1997) The ethics of clinical research in the Third World. *N Engl J Med*, **337**, 847–9.

27. **DeCock, K., Shaffer, N., Wiktor, S., Simonds, R.J., and Rogers, M.** (1997) Ethics of HIV trials. *Lancet*, **350**, 1546–7.

28. **Aaby, P., Babiker, A., Darbyshire, J.H.,** *et al.* (1997) Ethics of HIV trials. *Lancet*, **350**, 1546.

29. **Semba, R.D.** (1997) Ethics of HIV trials. *Lancet*, **350**, 1547.

Section 2

Methodological issues in the experimental evaluation of sexual health interventions

What is the role of theory in the development of interventions? What are the relative merits of different randomised designs? What outcomes are appropriate and how should they be measured? What other information needs to be collected within trials?

Chapter 4

Using theories of behaviour change to develop and evaluate sexual health interventions

Stephen Sutton

Introduction

Health behaviour interventions are increasingly being based on theories of behaviour change.[1] A recent review of randomized controlled trials (RCTs) of behavioural interventions in sexually transmitted infection (STI) and HIV prevention identified seven trials that met rigorous methodological criteria,[2] including use of laboratory-diagnosed STI/HIV endpoints.[3–9] In each of these studies, the intervention was based explicitly on one or more theories of behaviour change. The theories were used both to develop the content of the intervention and, in some cases, to derive measures for assessing intermediate outcomes. Focusing on STI prevention, this chapter will discuss the role of theory in the development and evaluation of health behaviour interventions. First, the rationale for using theories of behaviour change will be outlined. Then, one theoretical approach, the theory of reasoned action,[10,11] will be described, and it will be shown how the theory can be used to guide the development of an intervention. Although the discussion focuses on this particular theory, most of the comments are also applicable to other theories of behaviour change. Finally, the chapter provides a detailed discussion of a number of problems and issues that arise when using theories of behaviour change as the basis for behavioural interventions.

Rationale for using theories of behaviour change

The rationale for using theories of behaviour change to develop and evaluate interventions aimed at STI prevention is straightforward, and can be summarized in the following four statements:

1. Behaviour influences STI outcomes.
2. Therefore, interventions aimed at STI prevention need to change behaviour.

3. Theories of behaviour change identify the factors that influence behaviour.

4. Interventions should therefore target these factors.

Theories of behaviour change: the theory of reasoned action as an example

Theories of behaviour change, also commonly referred to as *social cognition models*, are causal models: they specify a small number of proximal determinants of behaviour, or in some cases, proximal determinants of transitions between stages of change. These proximal determinants mainly consist of *cognitions* (i.e. beliefs, attitudes, intentions); some theories also incorporate *skills*. Both cognitions and skills are assumed to be amenable to change. Although important differences between theories of behaviour change are discussed in a later section, it is not the aim of this chapter to describe each theory in detail. Instead, one theoretical approach, the theory of reasoned action (TRA),[10,11] is outlined. This has been widely used to study STI preventive behaviours. A version of this theory was used as the basis for the interventions in the AIDS Community Demonstration Projects, which were aimed at members of hard-to-reach populations at risk for STIs/HIV,[12,13] and Project RESPECT, a multi-site RCT designed to evaluate the effectiveness of STI/HIV counselling and testing.[4] The reader is referred to other sources for useful descriptions and comparisons of the main theories of behaviour change.[14–16]

Figure 4.1 shows a simplified version of the TRA. Intention is the central component. According to the theory, behaviour is determined by the intention to perform that behaviour (e.g. the stronger a person's intention to use condoms, the more likely they are to use them). Intention, then, is the most proximal determinant of behaviour and the single best predictor of behaviour. The strength of a person's intention is determined by two factors: their *attitude toward the behaviour* that is, their overall evaluation of performing the behaviour; and their *subjective norm* that is, the extent to which they think that important others, such as partners or friends, would want them to perform it.

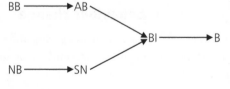

Fig. 4.1 A simplified representation of the theory of reasoned action. BB = behavioural beliefs; NB = normative beliefs; AB = attitude toward the behaviour; SN = subjective norm; BI = behavioural intention; B = behaviour

The relative importance of these two components may vary for different behaviours and different populations. Finally, attitude toward the behaviour is determined by *salient behavioural beliefs*, that is, beliefs about the personal consequences of performing the behaviour, and subjective norm is determined by *salient normative beliefs*, that is, beliefs about the views of important others. According to the theory, changing behaviour requires changing these underlying beliefs.

It is important to note that theories like the TRA do not rule out other causes of behaviour. Many other factors, such as socio-demographic, cultural, personality factors etc., are recognized as potential influences on behaviour, but these are assumed to be distal factors, in other words to be farther removed from the behaviour than the proximal factors specified by the model. The TRA is assumed to be *sufficient*: distal factors are assumed to influence intention only via their effects on attitude and subjective norm. Similarly, assuming that intentions are stable, and that the behaviour is completely under volitional control, the effects of distal factors on behaviour are assumed to be entirely mediated by attitude, subjective norm and intention. These assumptions are testable, at least in principle. For example, there may be ethnic differences in frequency of condom use. This would be entirely consistent with the TRA: the theory would explain this in terms of different ethnic groups having different attitudes or subjective norms, and hence different intentions, with respect to condom use. Thus, theories of behaviour change like the TRA divide the determinants of behaviour into two classes: a small number of proximal determinants, which are specified by the theory; and all other causes, which are left unspecified, but which are assumed to be distal, and to influence behaviour only via their effects on the proximal determinants. For a recent application of the TRA and its extension, the theory of planned behaviour (TPB),[17] to the prediction of condom use intentions, see a paper by Sutton *et al.*[18]

Implications for intervention

Theories of behaviour change have direct implications for intervention. A model such as the TRA can be regarded as one component of a larger causal model (Fig. 4.2). In the simplest case, the box at the top of the figure would represent a comparison between an intervention condition and a no-intervention control condition in a randomized between-individuals design. In this case, the box is a dummy variable representing the comparison between two groups. Arrows are shown from the intervention box to each of the components of the TRA. Path *a* represents the direct effect of the intervention on attitude toward the behaviour. Although it is shown as a direct effect, this path is assumed to be mediated by behavioural beliefs. In other words, if the

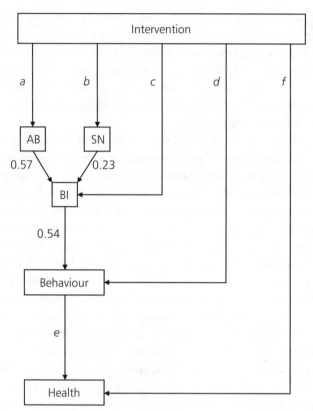

Fig. 4.2 Causal model for explaining the effects of an intervention on behavioural and health outcomes. AB = attitude toward the behaviour; SN = subjective norm; BI = behavioural intention

intervention influences attitude such that the mean attitude score in the intervention group is higher than the mean attitude score in the control group, then, according to the theory, this must be because the intervention has influenced behavioural beliefs. Similarly, path *b* represents the direct effect of the intervention on subjective norm, which is assumed to be mediated by normative beliefs. Paths *c* and *d* represent the direct effects of the intervention on intention and behaviour, respectively. Theoretically, these paths should be zero because of the sufficiency assumptions made by the TRA. Path *e* represents the effect of the target behaviour on the main health outcome: for example, the effect of consistency of condom use on the likelihood of becoming infected with an STI within a given time period. Finally, path *f* represents the direct effect of the intervention on the principal health outcome. The target behaviour for the intervention may be only one of a number of behaviours that influence the health outcome.

It is conceivable that the intervention may affect the health outcome by changing these behaviours instead of, or as well as, the target behaviour.

Drawing a causal model, such as the one in Fig. 4.2, is a useful early step in the development of an intervention.[19] The model is highly simplified, and it can, and should, be elaborated in various ways. The target behaviour(s) and health outcome(s) need to be specified. For particular behaviours and health outcomes, it may be possible to put numbers on some of the paths to represent the estimated size of the effects, and perhaps also the degree of precision attached to these estimates. Such estimates could be drawn from relevant primary studies or from meta-analyses. As an illustration, the numbers shown in Fig. 4.2 are taken from a recent meta-analysis, by Albarracin and colleagues, of 42 studies of the TRA and the TPB applied to condom use.[20] The numbers are standardized partial regression coefficients (beta weights), which can be interpreted as estimates of causal effects measured in standard deviation (SD) units. Thus, holding subjective norm constant, an increase of one SD unit in attitude is expected to be associated with an increase of 0.57 SD units in intention; and an increase of one SD unit in intention is expected to be associated with an increase of 0.54 SD units in reported condom use. As in many other behavioural domains, attitude was a more important predictor of intention than was subjective norm.

Such estimates may be helpful in planning and developing interventions. For example, they give an idea of how much attitude change an intervention needs to produce in order to yield the desired change in behaviour. This analysis could be extended by adding a coefficient to path e to represent the expected effect of the target behaviour on the main health outcome.

Currently, almost all the evidence from which such estimates could be drawn derives from non-experimental studies. For example, all the studies included in the meta-analysis by Albarracin et al.[20] employed a non-experimental design. Using such data to plan and develop interventions requires strong assumptions, namely that the effects are causal, and that the coefficients, (which derive from analyses relating observed between-individual differences in variable X to observed between-individual differences in variable Y), are accurate estimates of the effect on Y of manipulating X by means of an intervention.

Fishbein[21] argues that, although each behaviour is determined by the same limited set of variables (attitude, subjective norm, and intention, according to the TRA), each behaviour is also substantively unique, in two senses. First, for a given population or culture, the relative importance of attitude and subjective norm may vary across different behaviours. Second, for a given population or culture, the behavioural and normative beliefs that underlie attitude and subjective norm respectively may also differ for different behaviours. In the same way, for a given behaviour, the relative importance of attitude and subjective norm and the content of the underlying beliefs may vary across different cultures or populations. Fishbein argues that behaviours should be defined quite specifically, for example 'always using a condom for anal sex with a new sexual partner', and that the most effective interventions will be those directed at a single behaviour, rather than at multiple behaviours, or behavioural categories such as 'condom use'.

The originators of the TRA and the TPB emphasise the importance of using *correspondent* or *compatible* measures of the theories' components.[10,11,17] For example, if the target behaviour is defined as 'always using a condom for anal sex with a new sexual partner', the principle of correspondence or compatibility holds that all the measures should use precisely that wording. Using correspondent measures has been shown to maximize the predictive power of the theories. Proponents of other theories of behaviour change should consider employing this principle.

Decisions as to which behaviour(s) will be targeted in an intervention, and used to define behavioural outcome measures, should be informed not simply by psychological theory, but also by the known epidemiology of the relationship between behavioural risk factors and the principal health outcomes in the target population, which may be complex.[22] From an epidemiological viewpoint, it may be more appropriate to use a composite index based on several risk behaviours.[22] This is addressed further in Chapters 8 and 9.

One implication of the argument that each behaviour is substantively unique is that meta-analyses, such as the one by Albarracin *et al.*,[20] that combine studies on different behaviours and different populations, may yield findings that are too heterogeneous to apply to a particular behaviour and population (see Chapter 11). Indeed, that meta-analysis showed significant heterogeneity. Furthermore, researchers planning to develop an intervention targeting a particular behaviour in a particular population will often find that there are no relevant primary studies to draw on. In this case, it is necessary to collect data from members of the target population before designing the intervention. The steps involved in the process have been discussed in detail elsewhere,[23,24] and will be only briefly summarized here.

Having defined the target behaviour and the target population, the first step is to conduct a qualitative elicitation study to identify the modal salient beliefs, with respect to the target behaviour, in a sample of people drawn from the target population. Those beliefs that are elicited first in response to open-ended questions such as 'What do you see as the advantages of your using condoms with new sexual partners?' are assumed to be salient for the individual. Those elicited most frequently in the sample are designated the modal salient beliefs. The next step is to conduct a quantitative study in a second sample from the target population in which all the TRA variables, including the modal salient beliefs, are assessed using closed-ended questions worded according to published recommendations.[11] Analysis focuses on estimating the relative contribution of attitude and subjective norm in influencing intention, and on identifying the beliefs that best discriminate between intenders and non-intenders. The findings are used to decide: (a) whether the proposed intervention should target the attitudinal component only, the normative component only, or both components; and (b) which beliefs to target in the intervention.

In a subsequent study, designed to evaluate the intervention, measures of these key components should be included as intermediate outcome measures. Thus, theories of behaviour change like the TRA help both to identify the variables to be targeted in an intervention and to guide the selection of outcome measures.

Problems and issues

Although the rationale for using a theory of behaviour change is straightforward, the choice of theory is a more difficult issue. There are number of different theories that could be used, singly or in combination, as the basis for an intervention. It is true that there is substantial overlap between the various theories with regard to the components they specify as determinants of STI/HIV-preventive behaviour. For example, the construct of *self-efficacy*, the belief that one can perform a particular behaviour, occurs in a number of theories, including social cognitive theory,[25] protection motivation theory,[26] recent versions of the health belief model,[27] the health action process approach,[28] and the TPB, in the form of *perceived behavioural control*, which Ajzen states is synonymous with self-efficacy.[17] To give another example, the information–motivation–behavioural skills model incorporates the TRA within the motivation component of the model.[29] On the other hand, the theories of behaviour change differ from one another in a number of important ways, including: their range of application; their formal structure; the degree of complexity; the extent to which the theories themselves and the measures of their components are clearly specified; the amount of empirical support for the theories; and their predictive power.

Range of application and formal structure

Table 4.1 shows a simple classification of theories of behaviour change by range of application (general, health-specific, and domain- or behaviour-specific) and formal structure (stage vs non-stage theories), with one example

Table 4.1 Classification of theories of behaviour change

	Stage	Non-stage
General	Transtheoretical model	Theory of reasoned action
Health-specific	Precaution adoption process model	Health belief model
Domain-specific	AIDS risk reduction model	IMBM[1]

[1] Information-motivation-behavioural skills model

in each category. General theories, such as the TRA, are those that, in principle, can be applied to a wide range of behaviours, not simply health-related ones. Health-specific theories like the health belief model apply only to health-related behaviours. Behaviour- or domain-specific models have a still more narrow range of application. For example, both the AIDS risk reduction model and the information–motivation–behavioural skills model were developed to understand STI-preventive behaviour, such as condom use.[29,30] Stroebe (see Ref. 31, p. 27) states a preference for general models for reasons of parsimony: '... it is not very economical to continue to entertain specific theories of health behaviour unless the predictive success of these models is greater than that of general models of behaviour'.

It is important to distinguish between stage and non-stage (or *continuum*) theories.[32] These two types of theories have different formal structures and different implications for intervention. Stage theories assume that behaviour change involves movement through a sequence of discrete stages, that different factors are important at different stages, and therefore that different (*stage-matched*) interventions, should be used for people in different stages. The best-known stage theory is the transtheoretical model,[33] which has been applied to a wide range of health-related behaviours, including condom use.[34] The version of the model that has been used most widely in recent years specifies five stages: pre-contemplation; contemplation; preparation; action; and maintenance. Although it is the dominant stage theory in the field of health behaviour, the transtheoretical model suffers from serious conceptual and measurement problems and cannot be recommended.[35,36] Possible alternatives to the transtheoretical model are the precaution adoption process model,[37] which is a health-specific stage theory, and the AIDS risk reduction model,[30] which is specific to the domain of HIV/STI-preventive behaviour. The latter model formed the basis for the interventions in two studies[3,7] included in the methodological review by Stephenson *et al.*[2] However, in neither case was the intervention matched to participants' baseline stage of change.

In order to clarify how stage theories should be used, a hypothetical example will be outlined. Suppose a theory postulates that behaviour change involves movement through three qualitatively distinct Stages (I,II,III), and that factors *a* and *b* influence the transition from I to II, whereas factors *c* and *d* influence the transition between II and III. When using this theory to try to change behaviour, it is first necessary to classify the target sample into stages. This requires a good measure of stages of change. People in Stage I should receive an intervention designed to change factors *a* and *b*, and people in Stage II should receive an intervention designed to change factors *c* and *d*. It is necessary to keep track of stage transitions, so that when people have moved from Stage I to Stage II, they can be given the intervention designed for people in Stage II.

Although stage theories imply the use of stage-matched interventions, *all* psychological theories of behaviour change, including both stage and non-stage theories, can be used as the basis for *individually* tailored interventions. The TRA, for example, implies that individuals who have a low score on subjective norm, (i.e. they believe that important others would not want them to use condoms), should receive an intervention designed to increase their subjective norm. In contrast, individuals who have a low score on attitude toward the behaviour should, according to the TRA, be given an intervention designed to increase their attitude. Target behaviours can also be individually selected.

Degree of empirical support

Degree of empirical support is a key criterion for theory selection. Some theories, for example the AIDS risk reduction model, have been tested in only a handful of studies, whereas others, for instance the TRA and the TPB, have been extensively investigated and gained substantial empirical support.[20,38] Unfortunately, the vast majority of studies that have been designed to test theories of behaviour change, whether in the field of sexual behaviour or in other domains, have used observational rather than experimental designs. Drawing causal inferences from non-experimental data requires a number of assumptions, some of which are arbitrary and untestable.[39] We need more studies in which the different components of a theory are manipulated independently, and their effects on behaviour estimated. For example, suppose a theory holds that factors X and Y influence behaviour. The strongest test of this theory would be to manipulate X and Y in a factorial experimental design. In the simplest case, we would create two levels for each factor, that is low X vs high X, and low Y vs high Y. We would then randomly assign participants to the four cells created by the combination of these two factors, and measure behaviour. This design would allow the additive and interactive effects of

X and Y on behaviour to be estimated. Measures of X and Y would also be included as *manipulation checks*, that is to check that the manipulation designed to influence X actually did so, and did not have an unintended impact on Y. With the important exception of research on protection motivation theory,[26] remarkably few studies have attempted to test theories of behaviour change in this way. Furthermore, few empirical studies have directly compared two or more theories.

A study in which explanatory variables are independently manipulated can be thought of as a kind of intervention study. However, studies that evaluate health behaviour interventions are not usually designed with the aim of estimating the independent effects of the explanatory variables. Instead, they try to change several explanatory variables at the same time, with the objective of maximizing the intervention effect. Thus, most health behaviour interventions are *multi-component interventions*. For example, suppose a theory postulates that factors X, Y, and Z influence behaviour. In a multi-component intervention based on this theory, participants may be randomly assigned to a condition that aims to induce high levels of X, Y, and Z, or to a condition in which these factors are maintained at their pre-existing low levels. If a difference in behaviour is observed, this can be interpreted as evidence consistent with the guiding theory, especially if it can be demonstrated that the intervention influenced X, Y, and Z as intended. Mediation analysis can be employed to test the hypothesis that the difference in behaviour was mediated by differences in the explanatory variables.[40,41] Note that such an analysis requires the same assumptions as other analyses of non-experimental data.

Many health behaviour interventions are not simply multi-component, they are also *multi-theoretical*: they draw on two or more theories of behaviour change. Combining theories requires careful consideration and explicit justification. It may create conceptual confusion, particularly when it involves theories such as the TPB, that, on their own, are intended to provide a coherent and sufficient explanation of behaviour, or when incompatible theories, such as stage and non-stage theories, are combined. Bandura criticises this practice of 'cafeteria theorising'.[42] To extend the metaphor, some health behaviour interventions are 'cafeteria interventions'.

Predictive power and effective variance explained

As well as differing in the strength of their evidence base, theories of behaviour change also differ in their predictive power. General theories appear to have greater predictive power than health- or behaviour-specific theories.[31] Meta-analyses of non-experimental studies of the TRA and the TPB, applied to a range of different behaviours, show that these theories explain on average between 40 and 50 per cent of the variance in intention, and between 19 and 38 per cent of the variance in behaviour.[38] It is noteworthy that the meta-analysis of the theories applied to condom use referred to in an earlier section yielded figures for the percentage of variance explained that fell within these ranges.[20] Theories of behaviour change are often criticized in the context of sexual behaviour, for focusing on individual cognitions and behaviours and failing adequately to take account of the dyadic nature of sexual encounters (see Chapter 2). Nevertheless, the TRA and the TPB perform equally well in this domain as they do in other behavioural domains.

However, an important caveat should be noted. In the case of the TRA, for example, the estimates of variance explained in behaviour reflect the effect of intention, the variable that is assumed to be most proximal to behaviour. But, according to the theory, it is not possible to intervene directly to change intention. Interventions must be applied to the most distal variables in the theory, that is, to beliefs. Estimates of the percentage of variance in behaviour explained by the distal variables, or the *effective variance explained*, are rarely reported but appear to be much lower than the estimates given above.[24] For assessing the intervention potential of a theory *effective variance explained* provides a better basis than the proportion of variance explained by the theory as a whole or the proportion explained by the proximal variables. Effective variance explained should therefore be routinely included in published reports. Also useful are measures of effect size based on partial regression coefficients, as in the causal model in Fig. 4.2.

Although strong theories are generally to be preferred, it is important to appreciate that a theory that has weak predictive power may still be useful from a public health standpoint, if the predictor variables are modifiable through interventions that have a wide reach, and if it is reasonably likely that the observed associations are due to causal effects of the predictors on behaviour.

Degree of complexity

Theories of behaviour change also differ in complexity. The transtheoretical model, for example, includes fifteen different theoretical constructs, whereas the most widely used version of the health belief model includes five (perceived susceptibility, severity, benefits, barriers, and behaviour). Other things being equal, it is easier to translate the components of a simple theory into intervention modules or sessions that target these components than it is if a complex theory is used. However, theories also differ with regard to how clearly the components are defined, how precisely the causal relationships are specified, and the extent to which there exist agreed or recommended operationalizations of the theory's components. The TRA scores highly in this respect. By contrast, the health belief model and the transtheoretical model are not well specified. When reporting an intervention trial, researchers should provide a detailed description of the content of the intervention, and how this maps onto the components of the guiding theory and the intermediate outcome measures, so that readers can assess the fidelity of the translation process.

Changing the proximal determinants of behaviour

A major limitation of psychological theories of behaviour change is that they specify the factors that influence behaviour or, in the case of stage theories, the factors that influence stage transitions, but they do not, in general, specify how to change these factors. For example, the health belief model postulates that perceived susceptibility, (e.g. perceived risk of becoming infected with HIV if condoms are not used consistently), is one of the factors that influences behaviour, but it does not explain why people differ in perceived susceptibility, the factors that influence perceived susceptibility, or how perceived susceptibility can be increased. Similarly, the TRA does not specify how to change the beliefs that are assumed to influence attitude and subjective norm.

Researchers who wish to use a theory of behaviour change to guide the development of an intervention therefore need to draw on additional sources of information including their experience and intuition, relevant empirical evidence, and other kinds of theories, for example those drawn from the education field or theories of persuasion. The most widely used theory of persuasion is the elaboration likelihood model.[43,44] According to this approach, changes in beliefs and attitudes that are enduring, resistant to counter-persuasion, and predictive of behaviour, are most likely to be produced if a communication presents strong arguments, and if the recipients are able and motivated to think about and elaborate on these arguments. However, little research has been done on what constitutes a strong argument; empirical studies using the elaboration likelihood model rely heavily on pre-testing to identify strong arguments. Furthermore, relatively few studies have used the theory in the context of health behaviour change.[24]

There are many other aspects of an intervention that behaviour change theories cannot inform. For example, theories of behaviour change provide no guidance on: the ideal number or schedule of sessions; whether participants should be intervened with one-to-one or in small or large groups; whether role-play or audio-visual aids should be used; and so on. Thus, interventions can never be entirely theory-based.

Conclusion

Theories of behaviour change identify the factors that need to be changed in order to produce a desired change in behaviour.[1] This is the main reason for basing a behavioural intervention on a theory of behaviour change. A theory of behaviour change can be embedded in a larger causal model that specifies the hypothesized causal relationships between the proposed intervention, the determinants of the target behaviour, the target behaviour itself, and the main health outcome. Drawing a causal model with effect size estimates is a useful early step in the process of planning and designing an intervention. Such a model is also helpful in guiding the analysis of data from an intervention trial.

On its own, a theory of behaviour change cannot provide sufficient information to design an intervention. Given the substantive uniqueness of each behaviour, it will almost always be necessary to collect qualitative and quantitative data from members of the target population before developing the intervention. Among other things, such data can be used to estimate the relative importance of the different theoretical determinants of target behaviour in the target population. The findings from these studies can be used together with the guiding theory, other kinds of theories (e.g. theories of persuasion), other empirical evidence, expert opinion, intuition, and experience, to design the intervention.

Those who develop and evaluate behavioural interventions should be aware of the important differences between the different theories of behaviour change, for instance the distinction between stage and continuum models. The choice of theory should be justified in trial reports, and the process of translation from theory to intervention should be fully described in supplementary documents, so that readers can assess its fidelity.

Basing interventions on theories of behaviour change and developing them systematically should ultimately lead to more efficacious and effective interventions. However, before this goal can be achieved, the problems and issues raised in this chapter need to be addressed by researchers and practitioners. This will require more basic research on the theories themselves, on the determinants of risk behaviours, and on the relationship between these behaviours and STI outcomes.

References

1. **Rutter, D.R. and Quine, L.** (2002) *Changing Health Behaviour: Intervention and Research With Social Cognition Models.* Open University Press, Buckingham.
2. **Stephenson, J.M., Imrie, J., and Sutton, S.R.** (2000) Rigorous trials of sexual behaviour interventions in STD/HIV Prevention: what can we learn from them? *AIDS*, **14**(suppl. 3), S115–S124.

3. **Shain, R.N., Piper, J.M., Newton, E.R.,** *et al.* (1999) A randomised, controlled trial of a behavioral intervention to prevent sexually transmitted disease among minority women. *N Engl J Med,* **340,** 93–100.

4. **Kamb, M.L., Fishbein, M., Douglas, J.M.,** *et al.* (1998) Efficacy of risk-reduction counselling to prevent human immunodeficiency virus and sexually transmitted dseases. *JAMA,* **280,** 1161–7.

5. **The National Institute of Mental Health (NIMH) Multisite HIV Prevention Trial Group.** (1998) The NIMH multisite HIV prevention trial: reducing HIV sexual risk behavior. *Science,* **280,** 1889–94.

6. **Branson, B.M., Peterman, T.A., Cannon, R.O.,** *et al.* (1998) Group Counselling to prevent sexually transmitted disease and HIV: a randomised controlled trial. *Sex Transm Dis,* **25,** 553–60.

7. **Boyer, C.B., Barrett, D.C., Peterman, T.A., and Bolan, G.** (1997) Sexually transmitted disease (STD) and HIV risk in heterosexual adults attending a public STD clinic: evaluation of a randomised controlled behavioral risk-reduction intervention trial. *AIDS,* **11,** 359–67.

8. **Imrie, J., Stephenson, J.M., Cowan, F.M.,** *et al.* (2001) A cognitive behavioural intervention to reduce sexually transmitted infections among gay men: randomised trial. *Br Med J,* **322,** 1451–6.

9. **Orr, D.P., Langefeld, C.D., Katz, B.P., and Caine, V.A.** (1996) Behavioral intervention to increase condom use among high-risk female adolescents. *J Pediatr,* **128,** 288–95.

10. **Fishbein, M. and Ajzen, I.** (1975) *Belief, Attitude, Intention and Behavior: An Introduction to Theory and Research.* Addison-Wesley, Reading, MA, USA.

11. **Ajzen, I. and Fishbein, M.** (1980) *Understanding Attitudes and Predicting Social Behavior.* Prentice-Hall, Englewood Cliffs, NJ, USA.

12. **Centers for Disease Control.** (1996) Community-level prevention of human immunodeficiency virus infection among high-risk populations; the AIDS Community Demonstration Projects. *Mor Mortal Wkly Rep,* **45,** RR6.

13. **Centers for Disease Control.** (1999) Community-level HIV intervention in 5 Cities: final outcome data from the CDC AIDS Community Demonstration Projects. *Am J Public Health,* **89,** 1–10.

14. **Weinstein, N.D.** (1993) Testing four competing theories of health protective behavior. *Health Psychol,* **12,** 324–33.

15. **Conner, M. and Norman, P.** (eds) (1996). *Predicting Health Behaviour; Research and Practice with Social Cognition Models.* Open University Press, Buckingham.

16. **Fisher, J.D. and Fisher, W.A.** (2000) Theoretical approaches to individual-level change in HIV risk behavior. In: Peterson, J.L., DiClemente, R.J. (ed.) *Handbook of HIV Prevention.* Kluwer Academic/Plenum Publishers, New York.

17. **Ajzen, I.** (1991) The theory of planned behavior. *Organ Behav Hum Decis Process,* **50,** 179–211.

18. **Sutton, S., McVey, D., and Glanz, A.** (1998) A comparative test of the theory of reasoned action and the theory of planned behavior in the prediction of condom use intentions in a national sample of English young people. *Health Psychol,* **18,** 72–81.

19. **Campbell, M., Fitzpatrick, R., Haines, A.,** *et al.* (2000) Framework for the design and evaluation of complex interventions to improve health. *Br Med J,* **321,** 694–6.

20. Albarracin, D., Johnson, B.T., Fishbein, M., and Muellerleile, P.A. (2001) Theories of reasoned action and planned behavior as models of condom use: a meta-analysis. *Psychol Bull*, **127**, 142–61.

21. Fishbein, M. (2000) The role of theory in HIV Prevention. *AIDS Care*, **12**, 273–8.

22. Aral, S.O. and Peterman, T.A. (1996) Measuring outcomes of behavioural intervention for STD/HIV prevention. *Int J STD AIDS*, **7**(suppl. 2), 30–8.

23. Fishbein, M. and Middlestadt, S.E. (1989) Using the theory of reasoned action as a framework for understanding and changing AIDS-related behaviors. In: Mays, V.M., Albee, G.W., and Schneider, S.F. (eds) *Primary Prevention of AIDS: Psychological Approaches*. Sage, Newbury Park, CA, USA.

24. Sutton, S. (2002) *Using social cognition models to develop health behaviour interventions: Problems and Assumptions*. In: Rutter, D. and Quine, L. (eds) *Changing Health Behaviour: International Research with Social Cognition Models*. Open University Press, Buckingham.

25. Bandura, A. (1997) *Self-efficacy: The Exercise of Control*. Freeman, New York.

26. Rogers, R.W. (1983) Cognitive and physiological processes in fear appeals and attitude change: a revised theory of protection motivation. In: Cacioppo, J.T., Petty, R.E., and Shapiro, D. (eds): *Social Psychophysiology: A Sourcebook*. Guilford, New York.

27. Strecher, V.J. and Rosenstock, I.M. (2002) The health belief model. In: Baum, A., Newman, S., Weinman, J., West, R., and McManus, C. (eds) *Cambridge Handbook of Psychology, Health and Medicine*. Cambridge University Press, Cambridge, pp. 113–7.

28. Schwarzer, R. and Fuchs, R. (1996) Self-efficacy and health behaviours. In: Conner, M. and Norman, P. (eds) *Predicting Health Behaviour: Research and Practice With Social Cognition Models*. Open University Press, Buckingham.

29. Fisher, J.D. and Fisher, W.A. (1992) Changing AIDS risk behavior. *Psychol Bull*, **111**, 455–74.

30. Catania, J.A., Kegeles, S.M., and Coates, T.J. (1990) Towards an understanding of risk behavior: an AIDS risk reduction model (ARRM). *Health Educ Q*, **17**, 53–72.

31. Stroebe, W. (2000) *Social Psychology and Health*. (2nd edition). Open University Press, Buckingham.

32. Weinstein, N.D., Rothman, A.J., and Sutton, S.R. (1998) Stage theories of health behavior: conceptual and methodological issues. *Health Psychol*, **17**, 290–9.

33. Prochaska, J.O. and Velicer, W.F. (1997) The transtheoretical model of health behavior change. *Am J Health Prom*, **12**, 38–48.

34. Prochaska, J.O., Redding, C.A., Harlow, L.L., Rossi, J.S., and Velicer, W.F. (1994) The transtheoretical model of change and HIV prevention: a review. *Health Educ Q*, **21**, 471–86.

35. Sutton, S. (2000) A critical review of the transtheoretical model applied to smoking cessation. In: Norman, P., Abraham, C., Conner, M. (eds) *Understanding and Changing Health Behaviour: From Health Beliefs to Self-regulation*. Harwood Academic Press, Reading, UK.

36. Sutton, S. (2001) Back to the drawing board? A review of applications of the transtheoretical model to substance use. *Addiction*, **96**, 175–86.

37. Weinstein, N.D. and Sandman, P.M. (1992) A model of the precaution adoption process: evidence from home radon testing. *Health Psychol*, **11**, 170–80.

38. **Sutton, S.** (1998) Predicting and explaining intentions and behavior: how well are we doing? *J Appl Soc Psychol*, **28**, 1317–38.

39. **Sutton, S.** (2001) Testing attitude-behaviour theories using nonexperimental data: an examination of some hidden assumptions. *Euro Rev Soc Psychol*, in press.

40. **Baron, R.M. and Kenny, D.A.** (1986) The moderator-mediator variable distinction in social psychological research: conceptual, strategic and statistical considerations. *J Pers Soc Psychol*, **51**, 1173–82.

41. **O'Leary, A., DiClemente, R.J., and Aral, S.O.** (1997) Reflections on the design and reporting of STD/HIV behavioural interventions research. *AIDS Educ Prev*, **9**, 1–5.

42. **Bandura, A.** (1998) Health promotion from the perspective of social cognitive theory. *Psychol Health*, **13**, 623–49.

43. **Petty, R.E. and Cacioppo, J.T.** (1986) The elaboration likelihood model of persuasion. In: Berkowitz, L. (ed.) *Advances in Experimental Social Psychology (Vol. 19)*. Academic Press, New York.

44. **Petty, R.E. and Wegener, D.T.** (1999) The elaboration likelihood model: Current status and controversies. In: Chaiken, S. and Trope, Y. (eds) *Dual-process Theories in Social Psychology*. Guilford Press, New York.

Chapter 5

Stages in the development and evaluation of complex interventions

Irwin Nazareth

Introduction

Over the last few years, there has been a growing interest in the experimental evaluation of complex interventions to improve health.[1-4] Complex interventions are made up of many components that act both on their own and in conjunction with each other. Interventions designed to change sexual behaviour are typically complex. Examples of complex sexual health interventions, directed at patients, health professionals, the community, and health services, are listed in the Box 5.1.

This chapter explores a framework for the design and evaluation of complex interventions for sexual health. It includes a detailed description of the sequential phases for the development of a randomized controlled trial (RCT), using a model that, until recently, was only applied to drug evaluations. The use of such an approach to the evaluation of interventions in sexual health is discussed, with special reference to an RCT of a behavioural intervention to prevent sexually transmitted infections (STIs) among minority ethnic women from Texas, USA.[5] The approach is also illustrated by a hypothetical intervention to involve general practice nurses in the management of chlamydia trachomatis. Finally, some of the practical difficulties encountered in following this phased approach to the development of complex intervention trials are discussed.

Framework for trials of a complex intervention

The use of a phased approach for the evaluation of a complex intervention that leads to the development and evaluation of a new intervention presents specific difficulties. The sequential framework developed by the Medical Research Council Health Services Research Board, as described in their web

Examples of complex sexual health interventions

1. Interventions directed at patients

- Health promotion activities directed at patients at risk of STD
- Interventions using psychological approaches to change sexual behaviour
- Computerized decision support systems used to educate patients

2. Intervention directed at health professionals

- Intervention designed to improve health professionals detection, treatment and prevention of STD (e.g. chlamydiae)
- The use of facilitators to implement a management plan for STD in family practice

3. Intervention at the community level

- Health education programmes designed to encourage safe sexual practice

4. Group interventions

- Sex education in schools designed to encourage safe sexual practice and reduced teenage pregnancy
- Education of minority high risk women groups on safe sexual practices

5. Delivery of services and organizational issues

- Shared care between primary and secondary professionals for patients with HIV
- The use of electronic communication for managing STD between primary and secondary care

page: www.mrc.ac.uk/complex_package.html, involves a series of steps derived from the evaluation of drugs (Fig. 5.1). It begins with a theoretical, or pre-clinical, research phase and ends with a post-marketing surveillance phase. These are described in further detail below.

Theoretical phase

The first step in the evaluation of a complex intervention is to ascertain a theoretical basis for the effects that would be expected of the intervention. This is discussed in detail in Chapter 4. Briefly, before developing a sexual behaviour intervention, it is essential to explore the existing sociological and psychological theories relating to the relevant consumers, professionals, and organizations.

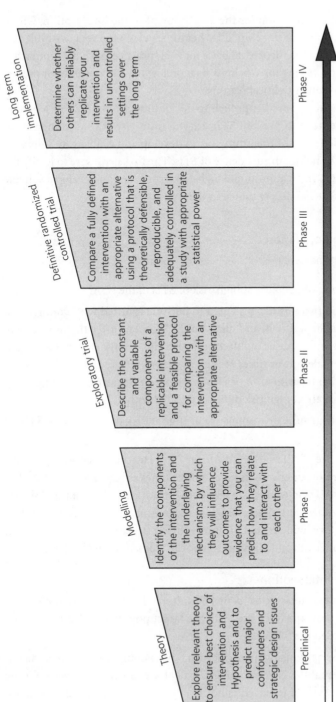

Fig. 5.1 Phases of RCT of complex interventions

Source: MRC April 2000.

This will set the foundation for the development of the intervention. Often, new interventions are developed by health service planners, without any attempt to explore the theoretical basis for such practice. Such an approach is unscientific; the driving force behind such policy may be consumer or professional needs, or other political reasons.

An example of a phased approach to development is an RCT of a behavioural intervention to prevent STIs among minority ethnic women from Texas, USA.[5] The aim of this study was to develop and evaluate an intervention designed to reduce the incidence of STIs. The first steps were to justify the need for an RCT in an appropriate high-risk group, and to develop a suitable intervention that was deeply rooted in theory.

Defining the population

Two key questions were posed:

1. Which group of people is at high-risk of STIs in the USA?

   Women are twice as likely as men to become infected with gonorrhoea, chlamydia, hepatitis B, and chancroid.[6] Women suffer the most severe symptoms and sequelae of infection with STIs.[7–10] HIV transmission from male to female is four times as high as that of female to male.[11] Rates of heterosexual transmission of HIV have been increasing,[11,12] suggesting that women are at high risk of being infected with STIs.

2. Which sub-groups of women are at higher risk of developing STIs in the USA?

   The incidence of AIDS amongst African- and Hispanic-Americans, as compared to white-Americans, is six and three times as high, respectively.[13] The figures for AIDS in women are seventeen, for African-American, and six, for Hispanic-Americans, times as high as white-Americans, respectively.[11,12] It was therefore evident that an intervention designed to reduce STIs in African-American and Hispanic-American women should be developed.

Defining the intervention

The obvious next step was to identify a suitable intervention that could be directly used, or adapted for use, with the target population. A review of the literature revealed the following:

1. Low success at reducing high-risk sexual behaviour among women due to sexual inequalities (i.e. women generally have less control over safer sex than men).[12,14,15] Moreover, minority ethnic women are at a disadvantage because of discrimination and disproportionate poverty.[8,14,15]

2. At the time of the study, only two published evaluations were identified, and none covered minority women.[16-18] This suggested a need to evaluate effective methods of reducing STIs in African- and Hispanic-American women. In the absence of a suitable intervention, the researchers decided to develop a new one, rooted in risk-reduction theory.

The intervention was primarily based on the AIDS Risk Reduction Model,[19,20] constructed on the basis of sound social psychological theory. The model also incorporated elements from: the Health Belief Model;[21] self-efficacy theory;[22] decision-making models;[23] and diffusion theory.[24] Information from the AIDS Risk Reduction Model, and from decision-making models, suggested that three stages of personal change are required before a person can reduce their risk of STIs: recognition of one's risk; commitment to reducing that risk; and following through that commitment by seeking solutions. The AIDS Risk Reduction Model had been developed for gay men. The challenge for the researchers was to apply this model to African- and Hispanic-American women.

Modelling (Phase I)

The next step in the evaluation of a complex intervention is to develop a suitable intervention, and an understanding of its possible effects (see Chapter 4). This requires exploratory work to identify the components of the intervention and the underlying mechanism by which these components influence defined outcomes in the population under investigation. A range of methods can be used during this phase, including surveys or other observational techniques, individual case studies and focus group interviews. To illustrate this phase, consider the hypothetical example of a study to involve general practice nurses in the identification, treatment, prevention, and follow up of chlamydial infections among women:

The intervention

The first step would be to define the component parts of the intervention (i.e. screening; treatment of women with chlamydia; provision of health education to prevent recurrence; and patient follow-up to ensure adherence to the management plan). Clarification of the components is best achieved by detailing the delivery of each part in a written manual, with appropriate action plans that are clearly described by diagrams or flow charts. If appropriate technology is available, the use of computerized decision-support systems should also be considered. Once these basic tools have been developed and approved, a training programme to assist nurses with the delivery of the intervention should be considered. Structured training is an essential pre-requisite to the success of the intervention, and requires careful planning. The application of appropriate educational strategies, such as interactive teaching and the use of role-play in addition to other traditional teaching methods, should be utilized. Good training ensures standardized delivery of the intervention.

Recruitment of patients

Before embarking on an RCT, it is important to estimate the approximate number of patients eligible to receive the intervention. Based on previous epidemiological research, the estimated prevalence of chlamydial disease in women in general practice is 2.6 per cent.[25] This would suggest that a practice nurse would have to screen at least 100 women in order to identify two or three cases. The acceptability and the costs of such an approach to case finding would need to be examined against other available options, such as screening a higher-risk group.

The outcomes

Selection of outcome measures should be based on a clear hypothesis. If we hypothesize that increased patient contact with the nurse will result in changes in sexual behaviour, and, eventually, in reduction in prevalence of STIs, then this hypothesized causal pathway should be reflected in the choice of outcome measure. This is discussed in detail in Chapters 8 and 9. Although the nurse-led intervention may lead to a reduction in the prevalence of chlamydial infection, any reduction is likely to be modest. Process changes, such as increased contact with health professionals, and behavioural changes, such as in sexual behaviour, are more likely to be observed. Thus, measurement of all these three outcomes would offer useful insights into the effectiveness of the intervention along the various levels of the hypothesized causal pathway, from early process changes to behavioural change, and clinical benefit (i.e. a reduction in chlamydia). The absence of significant changes in some or all of the three sets of outcomes would indicate the need for greater or lesser modifications to the intervention before further progress could be achieved.

Example: Application of phase one to an intervention of a behavioural intervention in women in the USA

The researchers in our example used the AIDS Risk Reduction Model,[5] which has been previously used in gay men.[20,21] However, the theory provided no guidance as to how one can accomplish movement through the three stages of personal change in the specific population of interest (i.e. African- and Hispanic-American women). Ethnographic data collection was required to adapt the AIDS Risk Reduction Model to the prevention of HIV and other STIs amongst these women.

A researcher conducted 25 focus groups and 102 in-depth interviews over 18 months with male and female African- and Hispanic-American people. These interviews explored conditions of life and lifestyles, values and beliefs, sexual behaviour, knowledge and concerns about STIs, including AIDS, perception of risk, relationships between men and women, drugs and alcohol consumption, condom use, strategies to motivate behaviour change and the logistics of intervention.[26] The resulting data provided insights into how to make the population recognize that they were at risk, and help motivate them to want to change their behaviour. These ethnographic research findings were then integrated into the AIDS Risk Reduction Model, with expert supervision and advice from a multi-ethnic team.

It was postulated that such an intervention would be expected to influence both behavioural and clinical outcomes. Hence, in the definitive trial, the researchers selected subsequent infection with chlamydia and gonorrhoea as their primary outcome measure, and change in sexual behaviour as their secondary outcome.

Exploratory trial (Phase II)

In this phase, all the data gathered from the previous phases is used to develop the best possible intervention and to guide the study design.

The Intervention

It might, for instance, be appropriate to vary the different components of the intervention, and to observe the effect this has on the whole intervention. In addition, the intensity of the intervention can be varied, just as different doses can be examined in drug trials. For example, in the case of the nurse-led intervention for chlamydial infection described above, we could limit the intervention merely to two components, such as the screening and treatment of chlamydial infection in women. Alternatively, the content of each component could be varied, for example screening by the general practice nurse and treatment by the general practitioner.

Another important consideration is the delivery of the intervention. It is known that the delivery of the intervention can change with time. In many cases, it improves as a result of a learning curve. But in other instances, it can deteriorate due to staff burn-out. It is therefore important to test for such changes over time. If a learning curve exists, the researcher might consider developing a run-in period before formal recruitment to the trial. Similarly, if staff burn-out is expected, an attempt must be made to refresh the intervention at an appropriate point in time. This can be achieved by revisiting the intervention and injecting a renewed energy into its delivery by addressing issues around health professionals' expectations and relevant organizational issues. The exploratory study can be used to assess the precise duration of the run-in time, or the stage at which the intervention might require a refresh-in phase. Often, burn-out might occur after several years of delivering the intervention, and this will only be identified in post-implementation surveillance, discussed below.

The exploratory study is also an ideal time to ensure whether the intervention is being delivered in a consistent manner. This can be achieved by techniques such as audio- or video-taping. In circumstances where privacy is essential, such as taking a personal history or conducting an intimate examination, direct observation by an expert would be more appropriate.

The control

The treatment of the control group must also be clearly described. This might include an alternative care package, standard (usual) care or no care. The last of these options is not often used in sexual or other health service evaluations for ethical reasons. Standard care and alternative packages of care, however, are commonly used, and vary in their complexity. Standard care, of any type, also changes with time. For these reasons, a clear description of the standard or alternative care package is essential in both phase two and three evaluation, using the same observational techniques employed to describe the intervention. If such observations were to suggest that standard care closely matched the intervention under evaluation, the researchers would have to redesign the intervention, or re-consider whether it would be appropriate at all to progress to a definitive trial.

Randomization

Exploratory trials should ideally be randomized for two reasons. Firstly, to examine the feasibility of random allocation, and, secondly, to allow for an assessment of effect size that would be used to calculate a sample size for the main trial.

Recruitment

The exploratory study provides an ideal opportunity to assess whether the expected levels of recruitment, as estimated during the theoretical phase, can be achieved in practice. The feasibility of recruitment within the clinical setting can also be assessed. It has been suggested that, before embarking on the exploratory study, researchers should set targets for recruitment over a specified time period. If the recruitment rate fails to reach these targets, the researchers would have to re-assess the recruitment process before progressing to phase three.

Acceptability of the intervention

The exploratory study must be used to assess the acceptability of the intervention to the professionals providing, and the people receiving, the intervention. Low recruitment rates might suggest poor acceptability. In such circumstances, the providers and participants should be interviewed in order to determine the acceptability, or otherwise, of the various intervention components. This can be done through one-to-one semi-structured interviews or focus group interviews. An analysis of the audio- and video- transcripts of the intervention, or of the field notes made by an expert observer, can also provide useful insights into the acceptability of the intervention components.

Example: Applying phase two to a study on sexual risk reduction

Details of the exploratory trial are not described in the evaluation report;[5] however, it is apparent that the following aspects of the study were developed from this phase.

1. *The intervention.*   Following the initial preparatory work, the intervention was developed and delivered over three sessions. Successive iterations of the three-session intervention were pre-tested with 13 groups (i.e. a total of 85 African- and Hispanic-American women). The content and objectives of each session were clearly listed and strictly adhered to by the facilitators, who were highly trained in the delivery of the intervention. Although the content was similar for the two ethnic groups, variations in cultural cues were emphasized. The sessions were standardized with scripts and flip charts. Random observations via one-way mirrors were conducted to ensure uniform delivery of the intervention. This process of refinement of the intervention facilitated the next stage of testing in a definitive RCT.

2. *The comparison group.*   These were provided with usual care, which was standard counselling. A detailed description of what comprised standard counselling was not, however, provided in the study paper.

3. *Randomization and recruitment.*   The process of recruitment and randomization was described in detail in the definitive trial report,[5] but it is unclear whether it was piloted. Much thought, however, had gone into the sequence of steps from recruitment to randomization, and it is likely that this was informed by an exploratory study.

Definitive RCT (Phase III)

This is the stage when an intervention is ready for a rigorous evaluation of its effectiveness. The main trial should address all the methodological issues posed by RCTs. Many of these are addressed in other chapters. In the case of the behavioural intervention trial to reduce STIs among minority ethnic women,[5] the preparatory work provided a sound basis for developing and refining an intervention that was rooted in psychological and social theory, and was relevant and sensitive to the needs of African- and Hispanic-American women. Thus, the stage was set for an evaluation of a complex intervention in a definitive RCT. The results of the study indicated a significant reduction in infection rates of chlamydia and gonorrhea (i.e. positive primary outcomes, in the intervention group, compared with the control group). Similarly, significantly fewer women in the intervention group than in the control group adhered to the treatment protocol, had multiple partners, or engaged in higher-risk sex (i.e. positive secondary outcomes).

Long-term implementations (Phase IV)

The purpose of this final phase is to examine the implementation of the intervention to practice, with special attention to uptake, the wider application of the intervention to other groups of people, the stability of the intervention; and the occurrence of any adverse effects. This will be achieved by long-term surveillance. Unlike drug surveillance, however, there are currently no existing mechanisms for this type of activity for evaluating complex interventions in sexual health. In order to achieve this, resources must be made available for a sufficient time period following the implementation of the new intervention.

This description of the sequence of progression through each phase is a simplification of a complex research process. In many instances, the progression is not linear but circular. Hence, if an exploratory trial suggests that a complex intervention is not acceptable, either to the professionals delivering it, or to potential recipients, the theoretical basis and components of the intervention will have to be re-examined. Nevertheless, it is necessary to do preliminary work in order to establish the active components of the intervention, so that they can be delivered as well as possible, and in a standardized manner, during the trial. Researchers must be able to offer a clear account of the detail of the intervention, describe how it influences various outcomes, provide a description of the stage of development (i.e. from theory to phase three), and describe recruitment levels, methods of randomization, the acceptability of the intervention, and the nature of the control group. This will eventually lead to the execution of an appropriately designed and relevant study.

Difficulties with using this approach in the evaluation of sexual health interventions

Until recently, RCTs have mostly been applied to drug evaluation. The increase in health services research over the last two decades, however, has led to an explosion in the use of this methodology.[1] Nevertheless, rigorous evaluation of sexual behaviour interventions is comparatively rare, and evidence of their effectiveness is only modest.[27] There could be various explanations for this. Researchers are often obliged to progress directly to Phase III or IV evaluations, because of inadequate time or resources for preparatory work, or because health service planners require the immediate implementation of a new service with rapid evaluation of effectiveness. Inevitably, many of these trials are unsuccessful, because of inadequate recruitment, inappropriate interventions, poor selection of outcome measures, and low acceptability of the intervention to the target population and/or the professionals. Use of an RCT may be difficult, for example, if people from the affected communities are involved in the planning and delivery of the intervention, or if the intervention is delivered via community networks or structures, or if it addresses socio-economic or legislative environments.[28] In such cases, a pragmatic approach to evaluation should take precedence over methodological purity.

Well-meaning attempts by sexual health researchers to adhere to a sequential phased approach have not been easy either, because of factors inherent in the topic under evaluation, or other external factors. The development of an intervention from an established theoretical base can present difficulties.[28] For example, the translation of sociological theories about sexual identity into a behavioural intervention can pose challenges at phase one. Securing funding from public and charitable grant bodies for pre-clinical work, or phase one or phase two evaluations, can also be difficult. Unlike drug research, commercial funding for preparatory work on complex interventions for sexual behaviour is almost non-existent. For example, although the Medical Research Council, one of the leading research funding councils in the United Kingdom, has endorsed a framework for developing and evaluating complex interventions in general practice, there is a total lack of clarity on how such applications will be funded. The application form, designed by the Medical Research Council Head Office for all clinical trial submissions, is exclusively designed for Phase III trial research. Nevertheless, the web document produced by the Medical Research Council (www.mrc.ac.uk/complex_package.html), is perhaps a first step in the right direction.

The methodology of complex intervention evaluation described in this chapter has been applied to a range of health service evaluations.

These include: educational intervention in primary care designed to change professional behaviour;[29] intervention in pharmacy practice designed to change medication-adherence behaviour in the elderly;[30] and brief psychotherapy interventions designed to improve depression in primary care mental health.[31] Despite the apparent diversity of these fields, the difficulties encountered by researchers in these studies are similar to those described here.

Conclusions

To enable a phased approach to the development and evaluation of complex interventions in sexual health or other fields, research funding bodies must commit adequate resources to detailed preparatory work. Research application forms should be structured to encourage researchers to follow this approach, and academic referees must be made aware of the principles underlying the design and development of new interventions in sexual (and other) health services. This might lead to a time lag from the generation of a new research idea to the completion of a definitive Phase III evaluation. However, it will result in fewer, but better designed and more relevant studies. The future of evaluative research in sexual health, based on the complex intervention model described in this chapter, will remain uncertain until there is a major shift in policy on the part of research funding bodies and health service planners.

References

1. **Campbell, M., Fitzpatrick, R., Haines, A.**, *et al.* (2000) Framework for the design and evaluation of complex interventions to improve health. *Br Medl J*, **321**, 694–6.
2. **Friedli, K. and King, M.** (1998) Psychological treatments and their evaluation. *Int Rev Psychiatry*, **10**, 123–6.
3. **Stephenson, J. and Imrie, J.** (1998) Why do we need randomised controlled trials to assess behavioural interventions. *Br Med J*, **316**, 611–13.
4. **Buchwald, H.** (1997) Surgical procedures and devices should be evaluated in the same way as medical therapy. *Control Clin Trials*, **18**, 1478–87.
5. **Shain, R.N., Piper, J.M., Newton, E.R.**, *et al.* (1999) A randomised, controlled trial of a behavioural intervention to prevent sexually transmitted disease among minority women. *N Engl J Med*, **340**, 93–100.
6. **Harlap, S., Kost, K., and Forrest, J.** (1991) *Preventing Pregnancy, Protecting Health: A New Look of Birth Control Choice in the United States.* Alan Guttmacher Institute, New York.
7. **Donovan, P.** (1993) Testing Positive: Sexually Transmitted Disease and Public Health Response. Alan Gutmacher Institute, New York.
8. **Eng, T. and Butler, E.T.** (1997) *The Hidden Epidemic: Confronting Sexually Transmitted Diseases.* National Academy Press, Washington DC.
9. **Wasserheit, J. and Holmes, K.** (1992) Reproductive tract infections: challenges for international health policy, programmes and research. In: Germain, A., Holmes, K.,

Piot, P., and Wasserheit, J., (eds) *Reproductive Tract Infections: Global Impact and Priorities for Women's Reproductive Health.* Plenum Press, New York.

10. **Aral, S.O. and Wasserheit, J.** (1995) Interactions among HIV, other sexually transmitted diseases, socioeconomic status and poverty in women. In: O'Leary, A. and Jemmott, L.S. (eds) *Women at Risk: Issues in Primary Prevention of AIDS.* Plenum Press, New York.

11. **Anon.** (1997) Focus on Women and HIV. HIV/AIDS Prev; July 1–2.

12. **Wortley, P. and Flemming, P.** (1997) AIDS in women in the United States. *JAMA*, **278**, 911–16.

13. **Wortley, P. and Flemming, P.** (1994) HIV/AIDS Surveillance Report. 6.

14. **Amaro, H.** (1995) Love, sex and power: considering women realities on HIV prevention. *Am Psychol*, **50**, 437–47.

15. **Acerbate, J., Wypijewska, C., and Brodie, H.** (1994) AIDS and behaviour: an integrated approach. National Academy Press, Washington DC.

16. **Boyer, C.B., Barrett, D.C., Peterman, T.A., and Bolan, G.** (1997) Sexually transmitted disease (STD) and HIV risk in heterosexual adults attending a public STD clinic: evaluation of a randomised controlled behavioural risk-reduction intervention trial. *AIDS*, **11**, 359–67.

17. **Kamb, M.L., Fishbein, M., Douglas, J.M.,** *et al.* (1998) Efficacy of risk-reduction counselling to prevent human immunodeficiency virus and sexually transmitted diseases. *JAMA*, **280**, 1161–7.

18. **Orr, D.P., Langefeld, C.D., Katz, B.P., and Caine, V.A.** (1996) Behavioural intervention to increase condom use among high-risk female adolescents. *J Pediatr*, **128**, 288–95.

19. **Catania, J.A., Coates, T.J., Kegeles, S.M., Ekstrand, M., Guydish, J., and Bye, L.** (1989) Implications of the AIDS risk reduction model for the gay community: the importance of the perceived sexual enjoyment and help seeking behaviours. In: Mays, V., Albee, G., and Shneider, S., (eds) *Primary Prevention of AIDS: Psychological Approaches.* Sage Publishers, Newbury Park, CA, USA.

20. **Catania, J.A., Kegeles, S.M., and Coates, T.J.** (1990) Towards an understanding of risk behaviour: An AIDS risk reduction model (ARRM). *Health Educ Q*, **17**, 53–72.

21. **Becker, M.H. and Joseph, J.G.** (1988) AIDS and behavioural change to reduce risk: a review. *Am J Public Health*, **78**, 394–410.

22. **Bandura, A.** (1977) Self-efficacy: towards a unifying theory of behavioural change. *Psychol Rev*, **84**, 191–215.

23. **Fishbein, M. and Ajzen, I.** (1975) Belief, Attitude, Intention and Behaviour: An Introduction to Theory and Research. Addison-Wesley Reading, MA, USA.

24. **Rogers, E.** (1983) *Diffusion of Innovations.* Free Press, New York.

25. **Grun, L., Tassano-Smith, J., Carder, C.,** *et al.* (1997) Comparison of two methods of screening for genital chlamydia infection in women attending in general practice: a cross-sectional survey. *Br Med J*, **315**, 226–30.

26. **Ramos, R., Shain, R.N., and Johnson, L.** (1995) "Men I mess with don't have anything to do with AIDS": Using ethno-theory to understand risk perception. *Midwest Sociol Quarterly*, **36**, 483–504.

27. **Stephenson, J.M., Imrie, J., and Sutton, S.R.** (2000) Rigorous trials of sexual behaviour interventions in STD/HIV prevention: what can we learn from them? *AIDS*, **14** (suppl. 3), S115–S124.

28. **Bonell, C. and Imrie, J.** (2001) Behaviour interventions to prevent HIV infection: rapid evolution, increasing rigour, moderate success. *Br Med Bull,* **58,** 155–70.

29. **Mason, J., Freemantle, N., Nazareth, I., Eccles, M., Haines, A., and Drummond, M.** (2001) When is it cost effective to change the behaviour of health professionals? *JAMA,* **286,** 2988–92.

30. **Nazareth, I., Burton, A., Shulman, S., Smith, P., Haines, A., and Timberall, H.** (2001) A pharmacy discharge plan for hospitalized elderly patients—a randomized controlled trial. *Age Ageing,* **30,** 33–40.

31. **Friedli, K., King, M., Lloyd, M., and Horder, J.** (1997) Randomised controlled assessment of non-directive psychotherapy versus routine general practitioner care. *Lancet,* **350,** 1662–5.

Chapter 6

Choice of experimental design

Sheila Bird

Introduction

This chapter considers the strengths and limitations of a range of evaluation study designs. It deals in most detail with the consumer principle of randomization. Although much of the chapter is devoted to randomized controlled trials (RCTs), non-randomized studies such as disease registries and cohort studies are included because of their importance in the evaluation of cost-effectiveness. The chapter also considers issues of informed consent that are relevant to choice of experimental design, and the need for database linkage to overcome informative loss to follow-up that might otherwise undermine randomized allocation.

An evolution of evaluation designs

The primary reason to randomize is for the comparison of interventions to be maximally unbiased.[1] Table 6.1 summarizes the strengths and limitations of an evolution of evaluation designs from RCTs with 50 : 50 randomized allocation down to non-randomized patient preference cohort studies.[2,3] It also includes examples of intentionally data-dependent allocation (play-the-winner randomization) and pre-randomization so that patients know the allocation to which they are being asked for consent (Zelen randomization).

Fairness in allocation of scarce resources is an incontrovertible reason for randomization, and informed consent is likely to be maximal—whatever the implied randomization ratio is. Preferential (but fixed) randomization ratio,[4] such as 60 : 40 in favour of a novel intervention, is uncontroversial; may enhance consent for randomization if patients reason that an RCT protocol which has passed peer-review, funders' and ethical scrutiny is likely to have at least an evens chance of making a treatment advance; and allows investigators to learn more quickly about the experimental treatment. More patients need to be studied than with 50 : 50 randomization but the increase is modest provided that the randomization ratio is not more extreme than 70 : 30.

The consumer principle of randomization[5] allows doctor/patient to choose to be randomized in the ratio 30 : 70 or 50 : 50 or 70 : 30; may thus enhance altruistic participation by patients who have a rational (or emotional) but uncertain preference; and also, choice of randomization stratum is a new, potentially informative patient covariate. But the consumer principle of randomization has never been applied, perhaps because it threatens both the (complete) uncertainty principle and equipoise, as discussed later; and it complicates analyses because choice of randomization stratum may drift during the accrual period, for example in response to published data from related RCTs.

So-called patient preference trials are those in which patients elect either for 50 : 50 randomization or for own-choice of intervention,[5] all patients who make an election having given consent for research follow-up. Their strength is that they maximize the number of patients studied; but, unlike the consumer principle of randomization, no unbiassed comparisons are possible between patients whose treatment, in addition to randomization stratum, was self-selected. Patient preference trials are unlikely to maximize the number of patients randomized. In essence, they offer patients a choice of three extreme allocations, namely 100 : 0 (absolute preference for treatment A) or 50 : 50 randomization (complete uncertainty between A and B) or 0 : 100 (absolute preference for treatment B).

Table 6.1 includes an evaluation design in which patients are randomized as to how the treatment decision will be made—*either* by 50 : 50 randomized allocation *or* according to patient preference. Consent has to be sought both for randomizing between randomized vs self-selected treatment; and for randomization between treatments A and B if the primary randomization assigned the patient to 'randomized allocation of treatment'. A separate power calculation is needed to ensure that this secondary randomization between treatments A and B recruits sufficient patients for the randomized comparison between treatments A and B to be powerful.

Play-the-winner randomization,[6] which has been adopted in practice,[7] adapts its randomization ratio as successes and failures accumulate on the rival treatments within the RCT. At its simplest, play-the-winner randomization begins with equal allocation between treatments A and B, represented by (say) 10A and 10B tokens. Thereafter, a success on A or failure on B adds a further A token to the pool whereas success on B or failure on A adds an extra B token. Each random assignment is made by drawing one from the pool of tokens at that time. Allocation, always random, adapts as successes and failures accumulate on the rival treatments. Adaptation may be group-sequential. One such scheme might be to assign the first 40 patients by 50 : 50 randomization, the second 40 patients by a randomization ratio which reflected the successes and failures of the first 40, the third 40 patients by a randomization ratio which

Table 6.1 Strengths and limitations of randomization and non-RCT evaluation designs

Design	Strengths	Limitations
Disease registry	Epidemiological—diversity of patients, treatments and practitioners. Sufficient number of patients. Longer-term effectiveness of treatments.	Restricted baseline, treatment and outcomes data, limited costs data. Potential reporting biases re whom to register and follow-up reporting. Treatment switches and side-effects often poorly documented. Informed consent for registration is often taken on trust by registries.
Research cohort	Research protocol for data collection. Sufficient number of patients. Longer-term effectiveness of treatments, and costs documented.	Often single-centre. Protocol re whom to treat (and how to treat) is likely to have changed over time, but changes may have been poorly documented.
Randomized controlled trial (RCT) with 50:50 randomization	Trial protocol & documentation. High quality data but limited time-horizon for outcomes and costs.	Sufficient patients randomized to establish short-term efficacy. Drop-outs from treatment or follow-up undermine RCT. Follow-up too limited for cost-effectiveness.
RCT with preferential fixed randomization ratio, such as 70:30	As above. Fixed preferential randomization ratio is uncontroversial, may enhance consent, minimal increase in number of patients to be randomized provided not more extreme than 70:30 randomization. Assigns more patients to experimental treatment about which there is more to learn and from which better outcomes are anticipated.	As above.
Consumer-preference among three randomization ratios, such as 30:70; 50:50; and 70:30	Allows consumer preference between rival treatments to influence choice of randomization ratio. All are randomized assignments, so that comparison between treatments is unbiased within	Threatens the (complete) uncertainty principle. Perceived as damaging to participation because randomizable patients are enabled to choose a randomization ratio

Table 6.1 (continued)

Design	Strengths	Limitations
	randomization stratum, and can be pooled across strata. May enhance altruistic participation by patients who have an uncertain but outcome-unproven preference. Choice of randomization stratum is a new, potentially informative patient covariate. Choice of randomization stratum is likely to shift as data from this and other RCT's accumulate; determinants of any important shift can be identified, e.g. centre, time or patient prognostic factors.	that differs from the equipoise represented by 50:50 randomization. Choice of randomization stratum likely to shift as data from this and other RCTs accumulate; and hence unbiased comparison may only be achieved if made within both randomization stratum and accrual period— for example, before and after interim results from a related RCT were disclosed in a conference presentation. Has not been put into practice.
Patient preference trials in which patients (consumers) are only allowed to choose between randomization extremes of self-selected treatment and complete uncertainty, represented by randomization ratios of 100:0; 50:50; and 0:100.	RCT complemented by documentation of outcomes for patients who rejected 50:50 randomization. Maximizes the number of patients studied.	Unlike above, no unbiassed comparisons are possible for patients whose treatment, as well as randomization stratum, was self-selected. May not maximize the number of patients randomized.
RCT of patients between 50:50 randomized allocation to treatments A & B; and self-allocation to treatment A or B.	Primary randomization means that similar patients are randomized to randomized (r) vs self-selected (ss) treatment assignment, so that any difference in outcomes between rA+rB and ssA+ssB must be due to how the treatment decision was made—by randomization or self-selection. Separate power calculation is needed to ensure powerful secondary, unbiased treatment comparison, which is between rA & rB.	Consent has to be sought both for RCT between randomized vs self-selected treatment; and for randomization between treatments A and B if the primary randomization assigns the patient to randomized assignment of treatment. Because two levels of consent are required, patients who could not tolerate 50:50 randomized allocation between A & B would not give consent to primary RCT,

Table 6.1 (continued)

Design	Strengths	Limitations
	Has been implemented in practice.	generalization from results of primary RCT depends on rate of participation in it by eligible patients. 50% participation rate would gravely undermine generalizability.
Patient preferred allocation, with informed consent for documentation	Consent, fixed protocols and documentation as for RCT may be improvement on registry and on research cohort data, both of which evolve.	Unbiased comparison is unavailable. Has been used in practice.
Play-the-winner randomization in which randomization ratio adapts as successes and failures accumulate on the rival treatments. At its simplest, begins with equal allocation between A & B, represented by (say) 10A and 10B tokens. Thereafter, a success on A or failure on B adds a further A token to the pool whereas success on B or failure on A adds an extra B token. Each random assignment is made by withdrawing one from the adaptive pool of tokens.	Allocation, always at random, adapts as successes and failures accumulate on the rival treatments.	Other aspects of patient preference than performance of the rival treatments are not taken into account. Early vs delayed failure, or different types of failure— such as intra-operative mortality vs return to chronic dialysis after renal graft failure—are not distinguished. Costs are not accounted for in adapting the randomization ratio, but could be.
Zelen randomization, in one version of which only those patients randomized to the experimental treatment are asked to give informed consent; alternatively, all patient are asked to give consent for the treatment to which they have been randomly allocated.	Removes uncertainty for patients who are asked for consent to treatment X to which they have been randomly allocated; rather than for consent to randomization between treatments X and Y. Unbiased comparison is between groups as randomized, **not** between consenters to pre-assigned treatments X vs Y.	Randomization as a basis for unbiased comparison between treatments X and Y is undermined if a notable proportion of patients pre-randomized to to X or to Y declines consent for the allocated treatment.

reflected the successes and failures of the second 40 patients and so on. Group-sequential adaptation can more easily take account of delayed failures than the fully adaptive play-the-winner randomization.

Consumer principle of randomization

The consumer principle of randomization allows a recruit to choose to be randomized in the ratio 70 : 30 or 50 : 50 or 30 : 70. An example sets the scene. For patients whose sexual behaviour puts them at risk of sexually transmitted infections, number of casual sexual partners and incidence of sexually transmitted infections in the past 12 months are prognostic factors for future vulnerability to sexually acquired infections. Behavioural risk and motivation to change are not necessarily aligned, however.

RCT is underway to compare an intensive behavioural intervention, involving six one-to-one 1 h weekly sessions with a counsellor, or a single-day group-session, attended by five patients for 2 h, which offers the benefits of peer as well as professional support. The alternative interventions require dramatically different inputs of counsellor time per five clients (30 h vs 2 h) and also deliver the contact differently: one-to-one over six weeks or during a single day for a peer group of five clients. Would you consent to 50 : 50 randomization?

Jim, middle-aged and bisexual, has a history of many casual sexual partners and high incidence of sexually transmitted infections. He is motivated to change his sexual behaviour, has tried unsuccessfully to do so before, dislikes group discussions, but likes the sound of the new intensive one-to-one sessions with a counsellor over six weeks as giving sustained encouragement. Eric, on the other hand, is in his early twenties, appreciates the opportunity for peer-group discussion, is at lower risk—he has had only one sexually transmitted infection in the last 12 months despite a number of casual sex partners—and, because he often works out of town, prefers a one-off 2 h session than to attend for six weeks.

The two men have different preferences. Neither wants 50 : 50 randomization. Both are prepared to be followed up after six months to find out about the impact of the intervention. Jim's preference for the more costly intervention cannot be accommodated outside of the randomized trial. In effect, without consumer randomization, Jim's choice was a stark 50 per cent or zero chance (by non participation) of meeting his preference. He therefore appreciated the opportunity that consumer randomization offered him to select 70 : 30 randomization in favour of the one-to-one counselling that he preferred. Eric well understood the importance of RCTs for robust evaluation of new procedures, and wanted to contribute despite his out-of-town working; but he was uncomfortable at having to choose, in effect, between a too low 50 per cent or unaltruistic 100 per cent chance of his preferred option by consenting, or not, to be randomized. With consumer randomization, Eric's decision was between 50:50 and 30:70 randomization to the 2 h group session, which was easier for him to attend and therefore preferable. The two men were interested and altruistic enough to want to know which was the better intervention, despite opposite personal preferences for one over the other. Both participated in the randomized controlled trial: Jim chose 70:30 randomization and Eric was prepared to be randomized 30:70 to a group session of the sort that many clinics offered as their standard intervention.

Equipoise[8,9] can result as the sum of opposite, systematic, perchance-misplaced patient preferences, such as by Jim and Eric in the above example. Preferences by later randomized patients may differ from those who were recruited early on, for example in response to more robust evidence on outcomes which has accumulated in this or other trials and which a revised patient information sheet is (or should be) informative about.[10] Compelling evidence is a reason for trialists to terminate randomization. Accumulating evidence, such as is reviewed by Data Safety Monitoring Boards (DSMBs), may (perhaps should) be reason for patients, doctors and trialists to consider a revised randomization ratio to other than 50:50.[11] Why do DSMBs so seldom alter the randomization ratio on emergent evidence, and in advance of conclusive benefit?

30:70 randomization is a perfectly valid randomization ratio for an individual clinical trial; and diverse individual trials with 50:50 or 30:70 randomization can be readily combined at meta-analysis. Likewise, it is perfectly valid, albeit unusual, for randomization ratio to differ between objectively-defined patient strata, such as: 70:30 randomization for clients at highest sexual risk; 50:50 randomization for intermediate risk patients; and 30:70 randomization for clients with low sexual risk as in the above example. Consumer preference for randomization ratio is a doctor–patient characteristic[4] which can be determined at baseline: and, even in conventionally randomized trials, either adjusted for at analysis or used to define patient strata to ensure that treatments are allocated evenly (conventionally 50:50) within strata as well as across the trial.

Tilting the randomization ratio in accordance with patient preference, such as 70:30 for patients who prefer the new, more costly procedure; 50:50 for those who have no strong preference; 30:70 for those who prefer the standard, brief intervention is a small scientific step for triallists, but a large step for consumerism.[12] Then, if doctor–patient preferences evolve as the trial progresses, this will be evident from the distribution of patients between randomization strata in the first vs last third of the trial.[4] Preference is an extra covariate which may be prognostic in its own right, or prognostication may depend on whether randomly assigned treatment accords (or not) with the patient's expressed preference.

The consumer principle of randomization has not been implemented in the eight years since it was enunciated. Why not? Slavish adherence to conventionally-randomized trials for fear of giving ground on the complete-uncertainty principle[8] seems to be the major reason. Patient-consumers, their physicians and families will need themselves to campaign for a choice of randomization ratios to be offered in order for triallists to be persuaded that there is a reforming agenda which they need to address. Data Safety Monitoring Boards, in particular, should look to their responsibilities to participants in RCTs by reviewing the appropriateness of 50 : 50 randomization at each scheduled interim analysis.

CONSORT guidelines for the reporting of RCTs[13,14] seek to know the proportion of eligible patients who consent to randomization as well as about post-randomization withdrawals from (a) randomized treatment or (b) trial follow-up. It remains to be seen whether the consumer principle of randomization can serve to increase the first without adding to the second. As Pocock and Elbourne remark,[15] only randomized treatment assignment can provide a reliably unbiased estimate of treatment effects. Even so, informative losses to follow-up and non-compliance may muddy the waters.[16,17] Consumer preference between randomized treatments is a baseline covariate that most triallists have shied away from eliciting because patients' responses may confound the uncertainty principle by exhibiting uncomfortable elements of rationality in preferences, such as in the cases of Jim and Eric.

Cost-effectiveness and study design

When considering the potential biases associated with each of the above designs, the distinction between efficacy and effectiveness[15,18] has to be kept in mind and also the realisation that treatment withdrawals are likely to be informative (about non-compliance, lack of perceived benefit, or denial of treatment preference). Missing at random is usually a simplistic assumption. Cost and effectiveness, as well as efficacy, of interventions may be relevant in the choice of evaluation design. Disease registries and cohort designs are included in Table 6.1 because of their relevance to evaluating the cost-effectiveness of interventions. Cost data are increasingly collected in association with randomized trials because health technologies have to demonstrate cost-effectiveness as well as efficacy to be recommended for the National Health Service. In chronic diseases, cost-effectiveness is typically evaluated over a longer follow-up period than was required for proof of efficacy. Consequently, most evaluations of cost-effectiveness are ultimately non-randomized even if they start with RCT data on short-term efficacy and costs. Registries' epidemiological strength is that they include a diversity and multiplicity of patients, treatments and practitioners, and careful analysis may allow inferences to be made about the longer-term effectiveness of treatments (e.g. hip prostheses). However, baseline risk factors and outcome data may be less rigorously defined by registries than is usual for randomized trials. Research cohorts have the advantage over registries that there is usually a local protocol for data collection which all members of the research team have agreed. Unlike randomized trials, treatment protocols for managing patients in a research cohort are likely to evolve over time but changes are not always rigorously documented.

Informed consent

Issues of informed consent, including those debated in Zelen randomization,[19,20] are relevant in the choice of experimental design. Cluster vs individualized randomization[21] should not be selected as a means of circumventing properly informed consent[22] by patients within the cluster, be it a school or general practice or prison or genito-urinary medicine clinic. Typically, there are two aspects to informed consent: consent for randomization and consent for documentation of outcomes to be notified to the research team, irrespective of whether the patient has consented to, or had the opportunity to consent to, randomization. Even in cluster randomized trials, there is a duty to inform patients about the nature of the interventions to which clusters have been randomized. Given this information, some patients may prefer to change practice to one where the general practitioners have received intervention training, for example in provider-led HIV partner notification.[23] See[21,24,25] and Chapter 7 for discussion of when to prefer cluster randomization. Study size and analysis considerations are a little more complex in cluster randomized trials.[26] Pairing of clusters, one of which is then randomly allocated to the intervention, has important drawbacks:[27] if one cluster in the pair drops out for any reason, information from both is sacrificed; and relative risk is not estimable if no outcome event occurs in either cluster.

Sexual health interventions may be multifactorial, which invites randomized factorial allocation of components of the intervention for optimal understanding of their relative merits. Theory marches ahead of practice, however. Factorial designs are not discussed further in this chapter.

Sexual health interventions also raise important issues about whose consent matters. Often, the intervention is orchestrated via the index patient but the analysis concerns the contacts of the index patient. Sexual (or injecting) contacts of patients with acute Hepatitis B infection are an example. Whose 'rights' are infringed if the index patient 'prefers' a conventional, sub-optimal approach to contact tracing which the intervention seeks to improve upon?

Feasibility of sexual health interventions may dictate that their implementation is on a practice or area basis, which leads to cluster randomization,[14] but the outcome of interest is new acute sexually transmitted infections. Non-participation by practices denies the opportunity of participating in research and possible prevention to future patients. Practices' consent obliges subjects to participate in public health research for which they may not have given explicit consent. The best should not be the enemy of the good when it comes to informed consent.

Database linkage to reduce informative loss to follow-up

Sexual health interventions are often targetted at marginalized patients who may be difficult to re-contact. Moreover, the beneficiary of the intervention may be the patient's sexual contacts rather than the index patient.[28] But, these contacts are accessed only through the index patient as intermediary: and so non-participation by the index patient denies potential benefits to contacts; consent by the index patient imposes randomization on contacts who have not given their informed consent. Index patients may have ethical reservations about their gatekeeper role, in much the same way that general practitioners[29] or schools[30,31] are the conduit for research teams' access to individual patients or pupils. Whenever there are potential difficulties in knowing in detail about individual outcomes of an intervention, whether for reasons of confidentiality, or reliance on an intermediary for re-contact, triallists should consider whether some form of non-nominal database linkage would allow surrogate outcome(s) to be measured in an unbiased way for all randomized patients. This mechanism should be explained to patients at the outset so that knowledge of it has been taken into account in their decision to participate.[32] Because the surrogate outcome is available for all patients, including those who do not return for follow-up, the informativeness of losses to individual follow-up can be gauged and adjusted for in analyses of individual outcomes.

An example of this is provided by two cluster randomized trials of school-based sex education interventions in Scotland and in England. The aim of both trials is to reduce the rate of unintended teenage pregrancy. In both trials, as a backup to repeat questionnaires about pregnancy history, trial participants can be linked to statutory notifications of abortion and live births. This follow-up mechanism is independent of whether the former pupil continues to respond to follow-up enquiries from the research team. (Database linkage for females is complicated by changes of surname following marriage, but this can be mitigated by additional linkage to the Register of Marriages).

Conclusions

There are alternatives to 50 : 50 randomization of participants in an intervention trial. Most of these accommodate an element of participant preference, while preserving the principle of randomization. Potentially, these designs could increase recruitment into trials, but they have not been widely adopted in practice for various reasons. In future, researchers should at least consider alternative randomization designs and methods of database linkage as a means of enhancing the validity of trials.

Postscript

This chapter has rehearsed many guises of randomization, some of them less familiar in practice than their elegance warrants. The consumer principle of randomization[4] was conceived as what I would have wished, some 20 years ago, for my late father's randomization in a colorectal cancer trial. Its reiteration in this chapter was inspired by the rationality of friends with breast cancer who confronted randomization.

References

1. Pocock, S.J. (1983) Futher aspects of data analysis, *Clinical Trials: A Practical Approach*. John Wiley & Sons, Chichester, pp. 211–33.
2. Silverman, W.A. and Altman, D.G. (1996) Patients' preferences and randomised trials. *Lancet*, **347**, 171–4.
3. Silverman, W.A. (1994) Patients' preferences and randomised trials. *Lancet*, **343**, 1586.
4. Avins, A.L. (1998) Can unequal be more fair? *J Med Ethics*, **24**, 401–8.
5. Gore, S.M. (1994) The consumer principle of rationalisation. *Lancet*, **343**, 58.
6. Brewin, C.R. and Bradley, C. (1989) Patient perferences and randomised clinical trials. *Br Med J*, **299**, 313–15.
7. Rosenberger, W.F. (1999) Randomized play-the-winner clinical trials: review and recommendations. *Control Clin Trials*, **20**, 328–42.
8. Weijer, C., Shapiro, S.H., and Cranley-Glass, K. (2000) For and against: clinical equipoise and not the uncertainty principle is the moral underpinning of the randomised controlled trial. *Br Med J*, **321**, 756–8.
9. Chaloner, K. and Rhame, F.S. (2001) Quantifying and documenting prior beliefs in clinical trials. *Stat Med*, **20**, 581–600.
10. DeMets, D.L., Pocock, S.J., and Julian, D.G. (1999) The agonising negative trend in monitoring of clinical trials. *Lancet*, **354**, 1983–8.
11. Jennison, C. and Turnbull, B.W. (2002) Group sequential tests with outcome-dependent treatment assignment. *Sequential Analysis*, **20**, 209–34.
12. Hanley, B., Truesdale, A., King, A., Elbourne, D., and Chalmers, I. (2001) Involving consumers in designing, conducting, and interpreting randomised controlled trials: questionnaire survey. *Br Med J*, **322**, 519–23.

13. Moher, D., Schultz, K.F., Altman, D.G., and Lepage, L. (2001) The CONSORT statement: revised recommendations for improving the quality of reports of parallel-group randomised trials. *Lancet*, **357**, 1191–4.

14. Elbourne, D.R. and Campbell, M.K. (2001) Extending the CONSORT statement to cluster randomized trials: for discussion. *Stat Med*, **20**, 489–96.

15. Pocock, S.J. and Elbourne, D.R. (2000) Randomised trials or observational tribulations? *N Eng J Med*, **342**, 1907–9.

16. Cox, D.R., Fitzpatrick, R., Fletcher, A.E., Gore, S.M., Jones, D.R., and Spiegelhalter, D. (1992) Quality of life assessment: can we keep it simple? *J Royal Stat Soc Series A*, **155**, 353–93.

17. Touloumi, G., Pocock, S.J., Babiker, A.G., and Darbyshire, J.H. (1999) Estimation and comparison of rates of change in longitudinal studies with informative drop-outs. *Stat Med* **18**, 1215–33.

18. Snowdon, C., Elbourne, D., and Garcia, J. (1998) Zelen randomization: attitudes of parents participating in a neonatal clinical trial. *Control Clin Trials*, **20**, 149–71.

19. Bjerkeset, O., Larsen, S., and Reiertsen, O. Evaluation of enoxaparin given before and after operation to prevent venous thromboembolism during digestive surgery: play-the-winner designed study. *World J Surg*, **21**, 584–9.

20. Zelen, M. (1990) Randomized consent designs for clinical trials: an update. *Stat Med*, **9**, 645–56.

21. Slymen, D.J. and Hovell, M.F. (1997) Cluster versus individual randomization in adolescent tobacco and alcohol studies: illustrations for design decisions. *Int J Epidemiol*, **26**, 765–71.

22. Medical Research Council. MRC Executive Summary: Personal Information in Medical Research. Medical Research Council, London: October 2000.

23. Mir, N., Scoular, A., Lee, K., Taylor, A., Bird, S.M., Hutchinson, S., Worm A.M., Goldberg D. (2001) Partner notification in HIV-1 infection: a population based evaluation of process and outcomes in Scotland. *Sex Transm Infect*, **77**, 187–9.

24. Hayes, R.J., Alexander, N.D., Bennett, S., and Cousens, S.N. (2000) Design and analysis issues in cluster-randomized trials of interventions against infectious diseases. *Stat Methods Med Res*, **9**, 95–116.

25. Campbell, M.J. (2000) Cluster randomized trials in general (family) practice research. *Stat Methods Med Res*, **9**, 81–94.

26. Yudkin, P.L. and Moher, M. (2001) Putting theory into practice: a cluster randomized trial with a small number of clusters. *Stat Med*, **20**, 341–9.

27. Simpson, J.M., Klar, N., and Donncor, A. (1995) Accounting for cluster randomization: a review of primary prevention trials, 1990 through 1993. *Am J Public Health*, **85**, 1378–83.

28. European Partner Notification Study Group. (2001) Recently diagnosed sexually HIV-infected patients: seroconversion interval, partner notification period and yield of HIV diagnoses among partners. *Q J Med*, **94**, 379–90.

29. Oakeshott, P., Kerrym, S., Hay, S., and Hay, P. (2000) Condom promotion in women attending inner city general practices for cervical smears: a randomized controlled trial. *Fami Practi*, **17**, 56–9.

30. Hart, G. and Wight, D. (1996) Ethical issues in setting up a randomized controlled trial of health education for children. The case of teacher-led sex education in Scotland. In: Oakley, A. and Roberts, H. (eds) *Evaluating Social Interventions*, Barnardos, London 1996.

31. Stephenson, J.M., Oakley, A., Charleston, S., Brodala, A., Fenton, K., and Petrukevitch, A., *et al.* (1998) Behavioural intervention trials for HIV/AIDS prevention in schools: are they feasible? *Sex Transm Infect*, **74**, 405–8.

32. Bird, S.M. and Rotily, M. (2002) On behalf of the late Dr A. Graham Bird and European Network for HV and Hepatitis Prevention in Prisons. Inside Methodologies: for counting blood-borne viruses and injector-inmates' behavioural risks, with results from European prisons. *Howard J Crim Justice*, **7**, 37–47.

Chapter 7

Cluster randomized trials of sexual health interventions

Richard Hayes

Introduction

Over the past five decades, the randomized controlled trial (RCT) has become one of the fundamental tools of medical research. In particular, evidence from RCTs is now recognized as a 'gold standard' for the evaluation of new health interventions. It is well accepted that the effectiveness of new biological products, such as drugs and vaccines, has to be proven in RCTs for licensing purposes. As discussed in previous chapters, there are equally cogent reasons why the impact of other types of health intervention, including programmes to promote sexual health, should be evaluated in rigorously conducted RCTs.[1]

In RCTs of drugs and vaccines, the products to be compared are usually allocated randomly to *individual subjects*. Individual randomization may also be appropriate for some RCTs of sexual health interventions. In many cases, however, it may be more appropriate to randomly allocate entire *clusters* of individuals to each condition. For example, depending on the design of the intervention, trials of behavioural programmes could employ randomization of schools, villages or entire districts. Such trials are referred to as *cluster randomized trials* or CRTs.[2]

In this chapter, we begin by discussing the rationale for employing the CRT design to evaluate sexual health interventions. Such trials require special methods for their design and analysis, that differ from those used in standard individually randomized trials, and we go on to briefly discuss these methods. Finally, we consider some of the limitations and disadvantages of this study design.

Rationale for cluster randomization in trials of sexual health interventions

There are five main reasons for adopting cluster randomization,[3] and we discuss each of these in the context of sexual health interventions.

Nature of the intervention

Some interventions are such that, by their very nature, they must be delivered to groups rather than individuals, and this is particularly common in the case of health promotion programmes. Two examples are mass media campaigns designed to promote safer sexual behaviour in the population, and school-based sexual health education programmes. In neither case would it be possible to randomly allocate the intervention to individual subjects. This contrasts with biological products such as drugs and vaccines, that are designed to be delivered to individuals. Community level interventions may be particularly attractive in programmes to modify sexual behaviour. Experience has shown that individuals are much more likely to change their own behaviour if they live in a community in which there is a general change in the *norms* of behaviour.[4]

Logistical convenience

In some cases, an intervention could be provided to specific individuals, but it may be logistically simpler or more acceptable to allocate it at group level. An example might be HIV voluntary counselling and testing (VCT) services. Such services are generally accessed by individuals, and testing and counselling is provided at individual level. However, in the context of a trial, it may be more convenient to randomly allocate certain communities to receive VCT centres, the other communities acting as controls. This may also be more acceptable to the population, especially in some developing country settings where the provision of a new service for some members of a community and not others would not be judged equitable.

Avoidance of contamination

Contamination occurs in an RCT when some subjects allocated to the control group receive the intervention, and vice versa. In a drug trial, this may occur if neighbours share medications, or if subjects sell drugs to other community members. Contamination may also occur in the case of sexual health interventions. For example, if chosen individuals in a community are given health education to promote safer sexual behaviour, they may discuss these messages with other members of the community. Further, if they adopt safer sexual behaviour, this may in turn modify the risk of others in the community who have not received the intervention. Randomization of entire communities is likely to reduce the degree of contamination, but may not remove it entirely, since there is always some movement and communication between neighbouring populations.

Capturing effects on infectivity

The fourth and fifth reasons for adopting cluster randomization are particularly relevant in trials measuring the impact of interventions on the transmission of *sexually transmitted infections (STIs)*, including HIV.[3] The individually randomized trial is well adapted to measuring the impact of a preventive intervention on the *acquisition* of infection by an individual subject, or in other words in assessing effects on *susceptibility*. However, some interventions are designed to reduce *infectivity* as well as *susceptibility*. For example, programmes for the prompt diagnosis and treatment of STDs are intended to reduce the sexual transmission of HIV both by reducing the susceptibility of HIV-negative individuals and also by reducing the infectivity of HIV-positive individuals. With the exception of trials in which sexual partnerships are studied (e.g. *discordant couple studies* where one partner is infected and the other is not), individually randomized trials are unable to capture the effect of an intervention on infectivity. Where whole communities are allocated the intervention, by contrast, the measured impact on the frequency of infection captures both effects.

Mass effect of an intervention

This is a related but distinct issue, and may apply even to interventions that have no impact on infectivity. When we intervene against a *non-communicable disease*, for example by providing drug treatment to hypertensives to reduce their rate of heart disease, the effect of the intervention is only seen in those who receive it. By contrast, when we intervene against an *infectious disease*, a benefit may be seen even in those who do not receive the intervention. For example, if a proportion of the population access improved services for STD treatment, this may lead to an overall reduction in the prevalence of STDs in the population. Even those who do not use the services may experience a reduction in STD incidence, because fewer of their sexual partners will be infected. This is an example of the phenomenon of *herd immunity*, which is well recognized in vaccine studies.[5]

Summary

It should be clear from the above discussion that the CRT design is appropriate for many, but not all, sexual health interventions. Each situation should be judged on its own merit, taking into consideration the criteria listed above. The individually randomized trial is likely to remain the method of choice for most biomedical interventions, such as vaccines and drug treatments. Even here, though, there are exceptions. For example, some vaccines are designed to reduce infectivity rather than to protect against acquisition of infection. And the Mwanza and Rakai STD intervention trials in East Africa,[6,7] which are described later in this chapter, were designed to test the hypothesis that the widescale provision of drug treatments to reduce population prevalences of STIs could bring about a reduction in the incidence of HIV infection.

The CRT will often be appropriate for health promotion interventions designed to modify behaviour. Sometimes both approaches are possible, and can be used to answer different questions. For example, the effects of counselling and testing services have been evaluated in individually randomized trials, in which individuals are allocated to more or less intensive modes of counselling.[8] Alternatively, if VCT services are provided at community level, a CRT design could be used to assess population-level effects of such services. Both designs have also been proposed for trials to evaluate the provision of safe services for male circumcision as an intervention to reduce the incidence of HIV and other STIs.

An additional strength of CRTs is that they are often able to provide data on the *cost-effectiveness* of interventions that are of considerable value to health policy makers.[9] By reflecting reductions in impact due to *incomplete coverage*, as well as capturing the added population-level effects discussed in section 'Capturing effects on infectivity' and section 'Mass effect of an intervention', the CRT comes close to mirroring the effect of an intervention programme as it would be applied in practice on a large scale.

Issues in design of CRTs

Definition of cluster

In designing a CRT of a sexual health intervention, careful consideration must be given to the appropriate definition of the *clusters* that are to be randomized. The clusters may be defined in terms of demographic, occupational or geographical units. These could be families or households, schools, or classes within schools, factories or other workplaces, medical practices, villages, arbitrary geographical zones marked off on a map, or larger geographical regions such as cities or districts.

Several issues need to be taken into account in deciding on the nature of the clusters. First, as discussed in section 'Nature of the intervention', the nature of the intervention may dictate the choice of cluster. For example, in evaluating the effects of a programme to train health clinic staff to provide a more youth-friendly service, the clinic would be a natural unit of randomization, the cluster corresponding to the catchment population of the clinic.

One of the reasons for adopting the CRT design, as discussed in section 'Avoidance of contamination', is to minimize the extent of *contamination* between the intervention and control arms. In the case of vector-borne diseases, such as malaria, this involves consideration of the natural *transmission zones* of the infection,[3] which in turn depends on the sizes of communities and the flight range of the insect vectors. In the case of STIs, the clusters may be chosen on the basis of information concerning sexual and social networks, so that the majority of sexual and social contacts occur within clusters.[3,10] Note that social as well as sexual contacts are often of relevance, particularly where there is concern over the diffusion or sharing of the information or attitudes that are disseminated through the intervention.

Statistical considerations dictate that, all else being equal, the more efficient design is one with a large number of small clusters, rather than a small number of large clusters (see section 'Sample size' for further discussion of sample size issues).[2] In practice, a compromise is often needed between the statistical requirement for many clusters, and the desire to minimize contamination by defining large clusters. Logistical and financial constraints also have to be taken into account. It may be more feasible to implement an intervention in a relatively small number of large clusters, rather than in a large number of smaller clusters, even if the total sample size is larger.

Three examples are given from developed and developing countries, all involving trials of health education to promote safer sexual behaviour.

Trial of peer-led sex education in secondary schools in England

In this trial, 28 secondary schools have been randomized to the experimental or control conditions. In the intervention schools, sex education is delivered by trained 16–17-year-old peers (from the same school) to classes of 13–14-year-olds from two successive year cohorts.[11] Control schools continue with their usual teacher-led programme. Effects on knowledge, attitudes, and reported sexual behaviour are being compared 6 months and 2 years post-intervention.

This intervention is delivered to entire classes, and so these could have been employed as randomization units. However, schools were randomized in order to reduce the contamination that would inevitably occur if different classes in the same age-group were in different arms of the trial, and for logistical convenience. The 28 schools are widely enough dispersed to preclude contamination due to mixing of students from the intervention and control arms. However, children in intervention classes will unavoidably have social contact with other children not covered by the intervention, including those in other age-groups in the same school as well as those attending other schools in the vicinity. A certain degree of contamination is therefore, impossible to rule out, and the trial may not fully capture the effect that would be achieved if the intervention was implemented throughout the school system.

Trial of community based sexual health interventions in rural Uganda

This is a three arm trial, in which the first arm receives a community-based IEC (information, education, communication) programme aimed at promoting safer sexual behaviour; the second arm receives the same IEC programme together with improved STD treatment services; and the control arm receives a general community development programme.[12] The cluster in this trial is the *parish*, consisting of several villages with a total population of about 15,000. Six matched triplets of parishes have been randomized to the three arms, and cohorts of adults from the general population of these parishes have been followed up over three years to measure the impact of the interventions on the incidence of HIV and other STIs.

While the IEC intervention could in principle be allocated at village level, health services are provided by clinics serving several villages. A cluster consisting of a group of villages, corresponding roughly to the catchment populations of clinics, therefore seems appropriate. This design choice also helps to reduce contamination, since there is considerable social contact between neighbouring villages, but less so between parishes. A further strategy to reduce contamination was to choose the study cohort from the three to five villages closest to the clinic, which is usually near the centre of the parish.

Trial of adolescent sexual health intervention in rural Tanzania

This trial combines features of both the English and Ugandan trials. The intervention comprises teacher-led peer-assisted sex education in village primary schools, combined with youth-friendly services for sexual health at local health units and community-based condom promotion and distribution. The randomization unit in this trial is the adminstrative *ward*, which typically comprises five or six villages, and a similar number of primary schools. Ten wards have been randomly allocated to the intervention arm and ten to the control arm. Impact on the incidence of HIV, STIs and pregnancy, and on reported sexual behaviour, is being measured in a cohort of around 9000 adolescents aged 14 years and older, recruited from the upper grades of all primary schools in each cluster, and followed up for three years.

Again the school-based programme could theoretically have been allocated to individual schools, although training, implementation and supervision of the programme are all facilitated by ward-level allocation. For example it has been possible for government staff at ward level to play a key role in the programme, as would be the case in routine implementation of the programme. This choice of cluster was also dictated by the health service component of the intervention, since each ward is only served by one or two health units.

Randomization at ward level also reduces contamination, since there is considerable mixing of youth between neighbouring villages. Finally, randomization of a large number of individual schools would have been logistically much more complex, and travel costs would have been greatly increased.

Matching and stratification

In an individually randomized trial, large numbers of subjects are usually randomized to the different arms of the trial. Randomization can generally be relied on to ensure that the treatment arms are closely similar with respect to risk factors for the outcomes of interest, even if these factors are unknown or difficult to measure, and this is one of the major strengths of this design.

In contrast, CRTs often involve randomization of a relatively small number of large clusters, and substantial imbalances in risk factors between intervention and control arms can occur quite readily by chance. Although it is possible to adjust for such imbalances in the analysis, the credibility and power of a trial will be greater if approximate balance can be achieved. There are a number of specific design options that aim to improve balance.

Matched pairs

The simplest approach is to group the clusters into matched pairs on the basis of their predicted risk of the primary outcomes of interest.[2,3] Within each matched pair, one cluster is randomly allocated to the intervention arm and the other to the control arm. Matched triplets and larger matched sets are obvious extensions for trials with more than two arms.

The aim is to match clusters on variables that are correlated with the outcomes of interest. Sometimes, data are available from each cluster on prior rates of the outcome. This provides a good basis for pairing providing the ranking of clusters on such rates is reasonably stable over time. An example is provided by the Tanzanian adolescent sexual health trial discussed in section 'Definition of cluster'. The final survey of the trial cohort involves measurement of HIV prevalence in adolescents aged 17 and over. Before the trial commenced, a population-based survey of HIV prevalence in adolescents of the same ages was carried out in each of the 20 study wards,[13] and used to rank the clusters with respect to HIV risk.

In other trials, no prior data are available. However, clusters can usually be characterized with regard to factors that are thought to be related to the outcome of interest. In the Ugandan trial, for example, parishes were grouped into matched triplets on the basis of geographical features that were known to be correlated with HIV prevalence.[12]

Stratification

The matched pair design is only effective if the matching variables are closely correlated with the study outcomes. If the correlation is poor, so that the variation in risk *within* pairs does not differ much from the variation *between* pairs, then pair matching may paradoxically result in a *loss* of study power.[14] This results because pairing reduces the number of *degrees of freedom* available for the statistical analysis.

An alternative, which preserves some of the benefits of matching while reducing the loss of degrees of freedom, is to group the clusters into larger strata and then to randomize *within* these strata.[2,14] This approach was in fact used in the design of the Tanzanian adolescent trial. The prior HIV rates in the 20 study wards, together with information on the geographical characteristics of the wards, were used to group the wards into three strata, assumed to be at high, medium and low risk of HIV (6, 8, and 6 wards, respectively). Half the wards in each stratum were then randomly selected to receive the intervention.

There is a consensus developing that, unless matching variables are very highly correlated with the outcome, stratification may be the preferred choice for CRTs with relatively small numbers of clusters. When there is a large number of clusters (say 50 or more), one can usually assume that an unmatched design will achieve adequate comparability.

Restricted randomization

A further refinement is to restrict the randomly chosen allocations to those which satisfy specified balance criteria. This preserves the benefits of randomization while eliminating the possibility of selecting by chance a configuration of clusters with poor balance.

This method was used to further improve balance in the Tanzanian adolescent trial. After grouping the wards into strata as described above, random allocation of wards to the intervention and control arms was restricted to those configurations satisfying additional constraints:

- Prior HIV prevalence in intervention and control arms equal to within specified limits

- Prior chlamydia prevalence in intervention and control arms equal to within specified limits

- Balanced representation of intervention and control communities in each administrative district. This was mainly done for reasons of political acceptability.

Sample size

Standard formulae for computing sample size requirements for clinical trials are well known.[15] However, special methods have to be used for CRTs. Observations on subjects within the same cluster usually tend to be *correlated*, and this means that a larger sample size is needed for a CRT to attain the same power and precision as an individually randomized trial.

A number of formulae have been published to assist with these sample size computations.[2,16] We provide a simple formula which can be used for an unmatched CRT with two arms (intervention and control) when the primary outcome is the *rate* of some event (for example, incidence of an STI or pregnancy):

$$c = 1 + \frac{f[(\lambda_0 + \lambda_1)/y + k^2(\lambda^2_0 + \lambda^2_1)]}{(\lambda_0 - \lambda_1)^2} \tag{7.1}$$

In this equation, c is the required number of clusters in each arm of the trial, and y is the person-years of observation in each cluster (assumed constant). The factor f represents the required power and significance level of the trial, and for significance at the five per cent level (two-sided test) we use $f = 10.5$ for 90 per cent power, or $f = 7.84$ for 80 per cent power. The assumed rates of the primary outcome in the intervention and control arms are λ_1 and λ_0 respectively. Finally, k is the estimated coefficient of variation (SD/mean) between the cluster rates in each arm of the trial.

Example

Suppose a CRT is to be conducted to measure the impact of a village-based health education programme on HIV incidence in a rural African population. A random sample of 200 initially HIV-negative adults is to be recruited from each village, and followed up over three years to measure HIV incidence. If we assume that 30 per cent are lost to follow-up, we can put $y = 200 \times 3 \times 0.7 = 420$ person-years per village.

Suppose that HIV incidence in the control villages is about two per cent per year, and that we expect it to vary from about one per cent to three per cent in most villages. Then we can assume the mean and SD of the rates are 0.02 and 0.005, giving a coefficient of variation k of about 0.25. We want to have 80 per cent power of detecting a 50 per cent reduction in incidence in the intervention arm. Then applying eqn (7.1), we require c clusters per arm, where

$$c = 1 + \frac{7.84[(0.02 + 0.01)/420 + 0.25^2(0.02^2 + 0.01^2)]}{(0.02 - 0.01)^2} = 9.0$$

suggesting that we require at least 9 villages per arm.

Note that y is the person-years of observation in the cohort of individuals that we follow up. We do not have to follow up the entire population of each cluster, and an alternative design option is to recruit a smaller cohort sampled randomly from the cluster population. This means that both y and c have to be chosen, and to assist in this choice it may be helpful to tabulate the required number of clusters for alternative values of y, k and λ_1.

For details of sample size computations for alternative types of study outcome (means or proportions) and for the matched paired design, the reader is referred to a more detailed account.[16]

Issues in statistical analysis of CRTs

Standard methods for analysing data from clinical trials assume that observations on all individuals are *statistically independent*. This assumption is invalid for CRTs, because as we have seen observations on subjects in the same cluster are generally *correlated*. This phenomenon is known as *intra-cluster correlation* and means that if standard methods are used to analyse CRTs, then p-values will be too extreme and confidence intervals will be too narrow.[2] In other words, the strength of evidence produced by the trial will be exaggerated.

These considerations mean that special statistical methods, that account for the intra-cluster correlation, are needed to analyse CRTs. Methodological work is still in progress on optimal methods of analysis in different situations. For a detailed account the reader is referred to specialized texts on CRTs.[2,17] Here, we briefly describe a simple method of analysis, which appears to be robust under a wide range of conditions,[18] and give an overview of some more sophisticated methods of analysis which are still under investigation.

Cluster-level analysis

The simplest method of analysis is to obtain a summary measure of the outcome of interest for each cluster, and to analyse these cluster results using Student's t-test, or a non-parametric equivalent such as the Wilcoxon rank sum test. Depending on the type of outcome, the cluster measure might be the *incidence rate* of some outcome (e.g. incidence of HIV infection in each village), the *proportion* of subjects with a defined characteristic (e.g. proportion using a condom at last sexual intercourse) or the *mean* of a quantitative variable (e.g. mean number of sexual partners during past two years).

Example

In an unmatched CRT of an adolescent sexual health intervention, it is proposed to use serology for *Herpes simplex* virus type 2 (HSV-2) as a biological marker of sexual risk behaviour. Suppose there are ten clusters in each arm, and that the observed seroprevalence rates of HSV-2 at follow-up are as follows:

Intervention clusters (%)	Control clusters (%)
12.5	18.3
15.3	13.6
9.6	24.1
14.7	19.9
20.5	17.0
9.1	12.4
11.5	22.3
14.2	16.5
16.5	19.0
10.3	20.3
Mean=13.4	Mean=18.3
SD=3.5	SD=3.6

Applying the unpaired t-test, we find that $t = 3.07$ on 18 df ($p = 0.007$), indicating that the difference between the arms is very unlikely to have occurred by chance. The difference in mean prevalence between the arms is estimated as 4.9 per cent ($=18.3-13.4\%$) with a 95 per cent confidence interval obtained using the t-distribution of $4.9 \pm 2.10 \times 1.6$ or (1.6 – 8.3%).

Although the assumptions underlying use of Student's t-test are unlikely to be fulfilled, especially where cluster sizes vary substantially, simulation studies have shown that the performance of this test is remarkably robust.

For matched pair trials, the paired t-test can be used in place of the unpaired test. The method can also be extended to adjust for imbalances in risk factors measured at baseline,[18,19] although this makes the procedure considerably more complex. In some circumstances, it may be appropriate to analyse rates or proportions on a logarithmic scale, in which case results can be expressed in terms of risk or rate ratios.

Regression methods

The simple methods presented in Section 'Cluster-level analysis' are sufficient for the analysis of most CRTs, and seem to work well even when there are small numbers of clusters. However they do have some limitations:

1. If we want to adjust for other factors (e.g. variables showing imbalances between arms at baseline), we can do this using a two-step procedure as mentioned above, but this is less convenient than a regression analysis in

which both cluster and individual level variables can be modelled flexibly in a single step of analysis.

2. Equal weight is given to each cluster, even though we may have much larger sample sizes in some clusters than others. We would in principle prefer a method that weights clusters according to the amount of information they provide.

A number of regression methods are available which meet these requirements, and which make allowance for the *intra-cluster correlation* of observations. These include *multilevel (random effects) models*, and *generalized estimating equations (GEE)*. The interested reader is referred to more specialized texts for further details.[2,17] Both methods can be fitted in standard software packages such as Stata (StataCorp, University Drive East, College Station, USA), and the fitting and interpretation of these models are very similar to standard regression methods (e.g. logistic regression for binary data). However, there are a number of potential difficulties with the fitting of these models and we recommend that expert statistical advice is sought before using them.

Despite their superficial flexibility and convenience, these models are based on a number of (complex) assumptions, and it is unclear how robust they are.[20] For trials with small numbers of clusters in particular, we would generally recommend use of the more robust methods based on cluster-level analysis as presented in Section 'Cluster-level analysis'.

Limitations of CRTs

As we have seen, the CRT may often be the method of choice for the rigorous evaluation of sexual health interventions. However, this design does have a number of limitations that need to be borne in mind by the investigator.

Replicability

An important aim of some CRTs is to obtain data on the effectiveness (and cost-effectiveness) of an intervention if implemented on a large scale, in order to assist health policy formulation. In reality, interventions in rigorously conducted trials are likely to be better resourced and implemented to a higher standard than would be possible under conditions of routine implementation. Thus, both costs and effectiveness are likely to be higher in a trial setting than when replicated more widely.

This is a general issue for RCTs, and applies even more strongly to individually randomized clinical trials of drugs and vaccines, which are usually designed to measure the *efficacy* of the product under optimal conditions of administration rather than *effectiveness* under routine conditions. However, an important component of cost-effectiveness studies based on data from CRTs should be *sensitivity analyses* in which likely effects on cost and effectiveness under different scenarios of practical implementation are explored.

Generalizability

To what extent can the impact observed in a CRT of an intervention be assumed generalizable to populations other than the one in which the trial was conducted?

This issue is relevant to all intervention trials. Even in clinical trials of drugs or vaccines, efficacy may vary due to differences between populations in the expression of disease or in host characteristics. However, generalizability is likely to be a particularly important concern in trials of sexual health interventions, both because the intervention itself may be difficult to standardize between populations, and also because the response to the intervention may depend on a wide range of cultural, social and biological factors. An additional consideration in CRTs of interventions against STIs is that the population level effects of mass implementation of an intervention may vary substantially depending on the underlying epidemiology of STIs in different communities.

These points are well illustrated by the results of two CRTs conducted in East Africa to measure the impact of STI treatment interventions on HIV incidence in the general population. In Mwanza, Tanzania, provision of improved STI treatment services through local health units was shown to reduce HIV incidence by an estimated 40%,[6] whereas in Rakai, Uganda mass treatment of the entire adult population for STIs had little effect on HIV incidence.[7] A number of explanations have been suggested for these discrepant findings,[21,22] including differences in the intervention strategies (periodic mass treatment vs continuous availability of effective treatment at clinics). There were also substantial differences in the epidemiology of HIV and other STIs between the two populations. In particular, the HIV epidemic was more mature in Rakai with a much higher prevalence than in Mwanza (16% vs 4%), and since the infection was distributed widely in the population it is likely that treatable STIs played a relatively more minor role in HIV transmission in Rakai.

It seems to be well accepted in the development process for biological products that new drugs and vaccines need supporting data from multiple trials before they are licensed for general use. Similarly, we should expect major health promotion strategies to undergo multiple trials. Ideally, these trials should be designed to be complementary, providing evidence on effectiveness in populations with differing epidemiological characteristics. In any case, the results of such trials need to be interpreted with some caution in view of these issues of generalizability.

Balance and power

As discussed in section 'Matching and stratification', the number of clusters randomized in a CRT is often relatively small. This may lead to imbalances between arms, and although adjustments can be made in the analysis, such imbalances may compromise the *credibility* of the trial. Thus one of the major advantages of randomized trials, that known and unknown confounding factors can be assumed similar across the arms,[15] applies only partially to CRTs when the number of units is small.

A further problem is that when designing a CRT, information is needed on the between-cluster variability of the outcome in order to do sample size computations.[16] Often, only limited information is available on this prior to the trial, raising concerns that if the variability turns out to be greater than expected, the trial may be inadequately powered. For this reason, assumptions made when determining sample size should generally be *conservative*.

Ethical issues

CRTs of sexual health interventions raise many important ethical considerations, but most of these also apply to individually randomized trials and observational study designs. A special issue raised by CRTs is the question of informed consent.[2] In an individually randomized trial, each subject can be fully informed of the objectives and design of the trial, and asked to consent individually to enrolment in the trial, random allocation to treatment arm, and prospective follow-up. In a CRT, entire clusters or communities are randomly allocated to intervention or control arms, and investigators need to consider who should give consent for this community allocation. While individual subjects can be invited for their consent for recruitment to study cohorts, and may be able to decline receiving the intervention (depending on the nature of the intervention), it is unlikely to be feasible for informed consent for community randomization to be obtained from all members of the community.

Conclusions

CRTs are generally substantial undertakings, often involving follow-up of many communities spread over a wide geographical area, over an extended time period. Because of the effects of between-cluster variability, they generally involve larger sample sizes than individually randomized trials. In view of their special design features, they need to be conducted by research teams with the necessary skills and experience. Such trials therefore tend to be expensive and time consuming.

In spite of their cost and complexity, and of the other limitations discussed above, CRTs are often the only way to obtain reliable evidence of the effectiveness of health interventions in circumstances where individually randomized trials are inappropriate. Several such trials of sexual health interventions have been conducted over the past decade. They have helped to provide rigorous data in areas where policy-makers were previously working in a vacuum, and their results have had a major influence on policy. The challenge is to ensure that CRTs are conducted when they are needed, and that they are carried out to the highest possible standards in order to maximize the benefit from the resources that are invested in them.

References

1. Oakley, A., Fullerton, D., and Holland, J. (1995) Behavioural interventions for HIV/AIDS prevention. *AIDS*, **9**, 479–86.

2. Donner, A. and Klar, N. (2000) *Design and analysis of cluster randomization trials in health research*. Arnold, London.

3. Hayes, R.J., Alexander, N.D.E., Bennett, S., and Cousens, S. (2000) Design and analysis issues in cluster-randomized trials of interventions against infectious diseases. *Stat Methods Med Res*, **9**, 95–116.

4. Rose, G. (1992) *The Strategy of Preventive Medicine*. Oxford.

5. Anderson, R.M. (1992) The concept of herd immunity and the design of community-based immunization programmes. *Vaccine*, **10**, 928–35.

6. Grosskurth, H., Mosha, F., Todd, J., *et al.* (1995) Impact of improved treatment of sexually transmitted diseases on HIV infection in rural Tanzania: randomised controlled trial. *Lancet*, **346**, 530–6.

7. Wawer, M.J., Sewankambo, N.K., Serwadda, D., *et al.* (1999) Control of sexually transmitted diseases for AIDS prevention in Uganda: a randomised community trial. *Lancet*, **353**, 525–35.

8. The Voluntary HIV-1 Counseling and Testing Efficacy Study Group. (2000) Efficacy of voluntary HIV-1 counselling and testing in individuals and couples in Kenya, Tanzania and Trinidad: a randomised trial. *Lancet*, **356**, 103–12.

9. Gilson, L., Mkanje, R., Grosskurth, H., *et al.* (1997) Cost-effectiveness of improved treatment services for sexually transmitted diseases in preventing HIV-1 infection in Mwanza Region, Tanzania. *Lancet*, **350**, 1805–9.

10. Wawer, M.J., Gray, R.H., Sewankambo, N.K., *et al.* (1998) A randomized, community trial of intensive sexually transmitted disease control for AIDS prevention, Rakai, Uganda. *AIDS*, **12**, 1211–25.

11. Stephenson, J.M., Oakley, A., Charleston, S., *et al.* (1998) Behavioural intervention trials for HIV/STD prevention in schools: are they feasible? *Sex Transm Infect*, **74**, 405–8.

12. Kamali, A., Quigley, M., Nakiyingi, J., *et al.* (2002) A community randomised trial of sexual behavior and syndromic STI management interventions on HIV-1 transmission in rural Uganda. *Lancet* (in press).

13. Obasi, A.I., Balira, R., Todd, J., *et al.* (2001) Prevalence of HIV and *Chlamydia trachomatis* infection in 15–19-year-olds in rural Tanzania. *Trop Med Int Health*, 6, 517–25.

14. Klar, N. and Donner, A. (1997) The merits of matching in community intervention trials: a cautionary tale. *Stat Med*, 16, 1753–64.

15. Pocock, S.J. (1983) *Clinical trials: A Practical Approach*. Wiley, Chichester.

16. Hayes, R.J. and Bennett, S. (1999) Simple sample size calculation for cluster-randomized trials. *Int J Epidemiol*, 28, 319–26.

17. Murray, D.M. (1998) *Design and Analysis of Group-Randomized Trials*. Oxford, New York.

18. Bennett, S., Parpia, T., Hayes, R., and Cousens, S. (2002) Methods for the analysis of incidence rates in cluster randomized trials. *Int J Epidemiol*, 31, 839–46.

19. Gail, M.H., Mark, S.D., Carroll, R.J., Green, S.B., and Pee, D. (1996) On design considerations and randomisation-based inference for community intervention trials. *Stat Med*, 15, 1069–92.

20. Donner, A., Eliasziw, M., and Klar, N. (1994) A comparison of methods for testing homogeneity of proportions in teratological studies. *Stat Med*, 13, 1253–64.

21. Fleming, D. and Wasserheit, J. (1999) From epidemiological synergy to public health policy and practice: the contribution of other sexually transmitted diseases to sexual transmission of HIV infection. *Sex Transm Infect*, 75, 3–17.

22. Grosskurth, H., Gray, R., Hayes, R., Mabey, D., and Wawer, M. (2000) Control of sexually transmitted diseases for HIV-1 prevention: understanding the implications of the Mwanza and Rakai trials. *Lancet*, 355, 1981–7.

Chapter 8

Biological, behavioural and pyschological outcome measures

Frances M. Cowan and Mary Plummer

Introduction

The aim of sexual health interventions is to reduce the adverse consequences of sexual behaviour. The outcome measures chosen to determine the success or failure of such an intervention will depend on the specific behaviours that the intervention aims to change, and the context in which the intervention takes place.

Essentially, outcome measures can be divided according to whether they are *externally measured* outcomes, for example HIV or sexually transmitted infections (STIs), condom sales, abortion statistics, observed sexual negotiation, or *self-reported* outcomes, such as age at first intercourse, condom use at last intercourse, attitudes and self-efficacy. While externally-validated markers are, at least theoretically, more robust (i.e. less prone to bias), all types of measures have their advantages and limitations.

In this chapter, we discuss the general points to consider when selecting outcomes for determining sexual risk reduction. In addition, we discuss the attributes, limitations, measurement, and interpretation of various biological, behavioural, psychological and other outcome measures of sexual risk reduction. The relationship of these different, but complementary, outcome measures with each other and with intervention objectives is discussed in the next chapter.

Points to consider when choosing outcome measures

An appropriate outcome measure is one that is robust, valid, acceptable, affordable, feasible to measure, and seen as relevant by affected communities, policy-makers and funders. It should also be an outcome in which there is likely to be a detectable rate of change as a result of correct intervention delivery.

Choice of primary outcome measure has a major impact on study design. Assumptions about the baseline prevalence and the likely change in this outcome measure form the basis of the sample size calculation for the study. It is clearly important to use a robust outcome measure to determine the effectiveness of an intervention, but if that marker has a very low prevalence in the population being studied, then statistical power may be insufficient to prove that an effective intervention is in fact effective. Given the complexity and cost of behavioural intervention trials, it would be difficult to overturn the results of an under-powered trial that showed no positive impact on the primary outcome measure. This could have lasting, detrimental repercussions for future funding and policy decisions. It is therefore important to consider whether the intervention should be deemed ineffective if this outcome does not change in response to the intervention.

In drug trials it is rare to determine response to therapy on the basis of just one endpoint. As long as the outcomes are pre-specified, and the sample size adjusted accordingly, it is possible to have more than one primary outcome measure. Alternatively, it is at least theoretically possible to combine multiple outcome measures to provide a composite score, although in practice this is difficult to do.

Ideally, multiple outcome measures are used to evaluate an intervention and assess its complexity. All measures have advantages and limitations, so the most valuable information is often obtained by using a combination, which determine the effectiveness of the trial objective in different ways, thereby offsetting the unique bias and measurement error associated with each individually. This technique is termed triangulation. Whether secondary outcomes are biological, behavioural or cognitive, they should be identified at the outset of a trial, as this helps to focus intervention development and implementation as well as providing statistical rigour. When selecting additional outcomes to measure, note that a study powered to detect changes in one outcome measure may be inadequately powered to detect changes in another.

An outcome measure is valid if it measures what it purports to measure. Determining whether a particular outcome measure is valid or not can be difficult. Outcomes that are externally validated are measured against an independent standard, which is deemed to represent 'truth'—the gold standard. However, as will be discussed in the following section on biological outcome measures, no assays are perfect, not even those deemed to be the gold standard, and 'truth' evolves. Establishing the validity of an outcome measure for which there is no external independent standard is even more difficult. Such measures are usually internally validated, by measuring the same outcome (e.g. age at first sexual intercourse) using a number of different measurement instruments. If the same response is collected using several different instruments, this is reassuring but could just imply *consistency* of response rather than *accuracy*. For example, a person might over- or under-estimate the number of lifetime sexual partners they have had, both in a face-to-face interview and when completing a questionnaire. The means of maximizing the validity of behavioural outcome measures is discussed further below.

The overall aim of the intervention is the most important determinate in selecting outcome measures. For a precisely focused intervention, measurement of the targeted behaviour or related biological markers is the obvious choice. For example, an intervention designed to increase condom use may assess the rate of condom use through condom sales records, recovery of used condoms, or reported use. In addition, since condom use is promoted to prevent acquisition of STIs and/or unintended pregnancy, measurement of changes in rates of STIs and/or pregnancy could also be used to determine intervention effectiveness. These biological outcome measures have the added advantage that they will only be affected by condom use if condoms are correctly and consistently used. However, as failure to use a condom does not always result in infection or pregnancy, a larger study will be required to detect statistically significant changes in rates of these biological measures than in rates of condom use per se.

For a less-focused intervention, such as an adolescent reproductive health intervention (ARHI) that aims to reduce the adverse consequences of early sexual activity, the choice of outcome measure may not be obvious. The context in which the study is taking place will be particularly important in choosing measures. It may, for example, be appropriate to determine the effectiveness of an ARHI in sub-Saharan Africa by its effect on HIV incidence. However, in Western Europe, where rates of sexually acquired HIV among adolescents are negligible, it would be more appropriate to measure events that occur more commonly, such as rates of chlamydial infection or unintended pregnancy. In either case, however, using a biological marker as the sole measure of effectiveness of the study would diminish the value of the study. Little information would be available on how the change was effected, for example, through delay in sexual intercourse, increased condom use, or reduction in number of partners. Triangulating the biological results with behavioural data can thus provide a wealth of useful information, which can subsequently be used to refine and improve the intervention.

The final choice of primary outcome measure will often be a pragmatic one, partly based on logistic considerations. For example, although a biological survey may be more desirable, researchers may be limited to behavioural research due to financial or technical constraints. Few behavioural measures, however, have been validated as surrogate measures of STI or HIV risk.[1] Peterman et al.[1] conducted an analysis of data collected from a randomized trial of a behavioural intervention that had collected both behavioural and biological outcome measures. The intervention was successful in reducing incidence of STI among participants. But they were unable to demonstrate that the behavioural outcomes used were good surrogate markers of STI risk, partly because participants appeared to act on HIV prevention messages to suit their individual circumstances. They found, for example, that people tend to have protected sex with risky partners and unprotected sex with safe partners.[1]

Biological outcome measures

Biological outcome measures suitable for determining sexual risk reduction include STIs (Table 8.1), Y chromosome, detection in vaginal secretions and pregnancy. Biological markers can be used to assess the relative risk of populations before the start of a study, in order to assess similarity between intervention and comparison populations. In the context of a randomized trial, biological outcomes allow an investigator to determine the change in rate of infection and/or pregnancy as a result of an intervention.

For the infections that can only be transmitted through sexual contact, detecting infection is evidence that the infected individual has been involved in sexual activity. It may also provide insight into the sexual lifestyle of the infected person's sexual partner and the sexual networks with which (s)he engages. An infected individual reporting one lifetime partner may be more at risk of further infection than an uninfected individual reporting five lifetime partners all of whom are

Table 8.1 Common sexually transmitted infections

Bacterial
Neisseria gonorrhoea
Chlamydia trachomatis
Haemophilis ducreyi
Treponema pallidum
Lympho granuloma venereum
Bacterial vaginosis
Calymmatobacterium granulomatosis
Protozoal
Trichomonas vaginalis
Viral
Herpes simplex virus type 2
Human papilloma virus
Human immunodeficiency virus

from a low-risk pool. For example, a 28-year-old woman who reports one life-time monogamous partner of eight year's duration may be deemed to be at low risk if quantitative behavioural data on her sexual lifestyle alone are collected (as often happens in questionnaire surveys). However, if she is infected with HIV-1 and herpes simplex virus type 2 (HSV-2), this indicates that her partner has engaged in high-risk behaviour, and that she may be at risk of further infection. This is the situation for many married women in Africa. Using number of lifetime partners to assess this woman's risk would be misleading. Only by collecting biological data, or more detailed behavioural data (which may be diffi-cult to do), can one confirm her increased risk. Conversely, a 23-year-old student who reports five lifetime partners, including two 'one-night-stands', but has no detectable evidence of infection, may be drawing her partners from a pool of low-risk men, such as students of similar age with very low rates of infection.

General considerations when selecting biological outcome measures

Type of biological outcome measure

Biological outcomes vary in characteristics such as transmissibility and curabil-ity. For example, some STIs, such as HSV-2, human papilloma virus (HPV), and HIV-1 are caused by viruses and are incurable. While people with these infections can be treated to resolve symptoms, the organism itself remains in their bodies for life. In contrast, STIs caused by bacteria, such as Chlamydia trachomatis, Neisseria gonorrheoa and Treponema pallidum (i.e. syphilis), can be successfully treated using appropriate antibiotic therapy. This means that the prevalence of bacterial infections in a population can be reduced by improving diagnostic and treatment services in the absence of any behaviour change. By contrast, there is no evidence that population rates of HSV-2 and HIV-1 can be altered by diagnosis and treatment of infected individuals, except by preventing deaths from HIV-1 and thereby increasing the overall population prevalence.

In populations where viral STIs are highly prevalent, as is the case for HSV-2 infection in many parts of Africa,[2,3] it may be difficult to detect significant changes in incidence over the duration of a trial if those with the most risky behaviours are already infected at the start. In this situation, these outcome measures may still be useful with adolescent populations that are just begin-ning to be sexually active, because not all of those at risk of infection have yet been exposed. In contrast, it is possible to detect new infections of the curable bacterial STIs among people who have been infected previously. Another type of biological marker of unsafe sex is a test that detects sperm DNA on vaginal swabs. This assay remains positive for fifteen days after unprotected intercourse, but has been shown to remain negative in consistent condom users, making it an attractive means of validating recent self-reported behaviour.[4]

Type of assay

It is possible to demonstrate evidence of an STI in two ways. The organism itself can be detected directly in the urine or genital secretions. Alternatively, antibodies to the organism (i.e. glycoproteins produced by the body's immune system in response to infection with that organism), can be detected in blood, saliva or urine. Interpretation of direct tests and antibody tests differ.

For assays that directly detect an organism, a positive test result indicates that the individual is currently infected. For curable infections, it is difficult to detect all incident (i.e. newly acquired) infections using these assays without very frequent sampling of the individuals concerned. Some new infections will be missed because of treatment or spontaneous resolution of infection during the sampling interval. In addition, in a cross-sectional survey, infections of long duration are more likely to be detected than those of shorter duration, although evidence on duration of these infections is poor. For example, it is not known how long it is possible to be infected with Neisseria gonorrhoea or Chlamydia trachomatis before natural resolution of infection occurs, or indeed whether this does always occur. For these reasons, tests that directly detect infection are more commonly used to determine prevalence, rather than incidence, of curable infections.

For assays that detect the presence of antibody to infection rather than the organism itself, a positive result only indicates that the individual has been infected with this organism at some point in their life so far. It does not indicate the timing of infection or, for infections that resolve, whether the individual is currently infected. This test result rarely becomes negative even after effective treatment of curable infections. As such, antibody testing of curable infections is used to demonstrate 'lifetime exposure' to the infectious organism. For both curable and incurable infections, by measuring the prevalence of antibody at two or more time points, such as at baseline and then sometime after intervention delivery, it is possible to determine the rate of new infections (i.e. cumulative incidence), during the sampling interval.

In the case of HIV infection, a means of detecting recent infection has been devised and validated, namely, the less sensitive enzyme-linked immunoassays (EIA) testing strategy, also known as detuned enzyme-linked immunosorbent assay (ELISA). Individuals with established infection test antibody positive on both standard-sensitivity and less sensitive assays. Individuals with recently acquired infection have low levels of antibody and therefore test negative on the less sensitive assay, but positive on the assay of standard sensitivity. The sero-conversion period detectable by the detuned ELISA has been defined for HIV-1 Clade B, such that subjects testing positive on the standard-sensitivity EIA (optical density >0.75), but negative on the less sensitive EIA (optical density ≤0.75) have, on average, sero converted within the previous 129 days, with a 95 per cent confidence interval of 109–149 days.[5] Work is underway to try and extend the sero conversion period that is detectable using an even less sensitive testing strategy, or by testing for low avidity antibody, a different technique that has been used to detect recent sero conversion of other viral infections. Clearly, these techniques have important implications for the design of behavioural intervention trials, as it is possible to measure incident HIV infection as an end-point at a single time point rather than by repeated measures over time.

It is theoretically possible to detect all STIs both directly and by detecting antibodies. However, in reality, direct and antibody assays that are sensitive and specific are not available for all infections. Details of some of the available assays for detecting antibodies and specific infections are given in Table 8.2.

Table 8.2 Some of the laboratory assays available for measuring biological outcomes grouped according to specimen required

	Available assays	Performance characteristics	Storage and processing	Notes
		SERUM		
Antibody tests				
HIV-1 and 2	ELISA, rapid point of care tests, particle agglutination assays, western blot	Excellent[30]	Transport at +4 °C. Store −20 °C	Detect lifetime exposure Serial testing can be used to determine
Herpes simplex virus type 2	ELISA, EIAs, monoclonal antibody blocking tests, western blot	Variable[31]	Transport at +4 °C Store −20 °C	incidence of infection
Trichomonas vaginalis	EIA	[32]Not well-established yet	Transport at +4 °C Store −20 °C	
Chlamydia trachomatis	ELISA and DIF	Variable[33]	Transport at +4 °C Store −20 °C	Some of the available tests discriminate poorly between C trachomatis and C pneumonia

Table 8.2 (continued)

	Available assays	Performance characteristics	Storage and processing	Notes
Neisseria gonorrhoea	CFT, EIA, IF, HA	Poor[34]		Limited utility
Haemophilus ducreyi	EIA	[35,36]		Lifetime exposure
Calymmato-bacterium granulomatis	Indirect IF	High[37]		Lifetime exposure
Other tests				
Less sensitive EIA for HIV (detuned assay)	ELISA	[5]Varies by HIV subtype	Transport at +4°C Store −80°C	Detects recent infection Validated for for HIV Clades B and E
Syphilis serology	Treponemal Enzyme Immuno Assays Non-treponemal antibody tests (VDRL/RPR) Treponemal Antibody test (TPHA)	[38,48]Good	Transport at +4°C Store −20°C	Poorly predictive in early infection
HIV RNA testing	Quantitative PCR	[40]Varies by HIV subtype		To determine effect of interventions designed to improve adherence
CD4 testing	Flow cytometry and others	[41]Choice of method depends on laboratory facilities available	Whole blood required Transport at room temperature Analyse within 48 h	
In development				
HIV avidity testing			Transport at +4°C Store −80°C	Detects recent HIV infection

Table 8.2 (continued)

	Available assays	Performance characteristics	Storage and processing	Notes
		URINE		
Antibody tests				
HIV-1 and 2	ELISA, Particle agglutination assays, western blot	High,[30] but less good than serum	Transport at +4°C. Addition of boric acid prevents bacterial overgrowth Store at +4°C, test within 6 months	Detects lifetime exposure Serial testing can be used to determine incidence of infection
Direct detection of organism				
Trichomonas vaginalis	Microscopy and culture	High for culture	First void urine (15 ml), use spun deposit	Leukoesterase dipstick test (LE) may be used to determine who to screen in certain populations[41]
Trichomonas vaginalis	PCR	High	First void urine (15 ml)	
Chlamydia trachomatis	LCR or PCR	High[43]	Transport at +4°C	Can pool specimens for PCR testing in low prevalence settings to reduce cost[42]
Neisseria gonorrhoea	LCR or PCR	High[43,44]	Addition of boric acid prevents bacterial overgrowth. Store at −80°C.	

Table 8.2 (continued)

	Available assays	Performance characteristics	Storage and processing	Notes
Neiserria gonorrheoae	Microscopy and culture[45]	Higher in men than women	First void urine (15 ml) Use spun deposit	
Other tests				
βHCG	Early morning specimen most sensitive	High	Transport at +4°C Store at −80°C	Detects pregnancy
In development				
HSV-2 antibody assay			Transport at +4°C Store at −80°C	

		SALIVA		
Antibody test				
HIV-1 and 2	ELISA, Particle agglutination assays, western blot	High,[30] but less good than serum	Use saliva collection device with preservative. Transport and store at room temperature	Detects lifetime exposure Serial testing can be used to determine incidence of infection
In development				
HSV-2 antibody assay				

		GENITAL SWABS (VAGINAL/URETHERAL/GENITAL ULCER)		
Direct detection of organism				
Trichomonas vaginalis	Microscopy and culture EIA	High[46] for culture, variable for EIA.	Wet preparation for microscopy. TV culture medium or TV In Pouch. Transport at room temperature.	
Trichomonas vaginalis	PCR	High[46,47]	Transport at +4°C Store at −80°C	

Table 8.2 (continued)

	Available assays	Performance characteristics	Storage and processing	Notes
Chlamydia trachomatis	LCR or PCR	High[43,47,48]	Transport at +4°C Store at −80°C	Can pool specimens in low prevalence settings to reduce costs[49]
Chlamydia trachomatis	DFA EIA	Less sensitive than DNA amplification techniques[41,50]	Non wooden swabs, sample must include host cells, transport at 2–8°C	
Neisseria gonorrhoea	LCR or PCR	High[43,44,47,48]	Transport at +4°C Store at −80°C	
Neisseria gonorrhoea	Culture	Less sensitive than DNA amplification techniques[50]	Selective transport media, incubate at 35–37°C in CO_2 enriched atmosphere	
HSV-2	PCR	High[51]	Transport at +4°C Store at −80°C	
HSV-2	Culture	High–less sensitive than PCR[51]	Transport at +4°C Store at −80°C	
HIV RNA		Dependent on specimen collection technique	Cervicovaginal lavage/swabs in women Semen in men	Quatification requires exact quantity of specimen to be standardised
Human Papilloma Virus	PCR	High[47]	Transport at +4°C Store at −80°C	

Table 8.2 (continued)

	Available assays	Performance characteristics	Storage and processing	Notes
Other tests				
Genital ulcer aetiology	Multiplex PCR	See ref 52		No commercial kit available, therefore requirement to develop in house assay
Y chromosome detection	PCR	See ref 4		To validate self-reported behaviour and condom use up to 15 days after intercourse
In development				
Point of care tests for CT and NG				Existing commercially available rapid tests of poor sensitivity and specificity

CFT: Complement fixation test; EIA: Enzyme immunoassay; ELISA: Enzyme linked immunosorbent assay; DFA: Direct Fluorescent antibody test; HA: Haemaglutination; IF: Immunofluoresence; LCR: Ligase chain reaction; PCR: Polymerase chain reaction.

Sample required

Which biological specimens need to be collected will depend on which infection is to be detected, which type of assay is to be used, the local study setting and available laboratory facilities. Specimens can include venous blood, capillary blood, dried blood spots, saliva, cervico-vaginal secretions, rectal secretions or urine, urethral secretions, and genital ulcer exudate. Less invasive methods of specimen collection, such as those for saliva or urine, may be more acceptable to participants and have higher response rates than relatively invasive methods, such as those requiring venepuncture or vaginal penetration. Similarly, the acceptability of a method may be affected by whether it is self-administered or not. For example, studies have shown that, in some settings, women can be trained to take their own vaginal swabs, or to collect vaginal samples using tampons. Women may find this more acceptable than undergoing genital examination by a professional.[6] However, a disadvantage of this form of specimen collection is that it may be difficult to standardize.

With the increasing availability of nucleic acid amplification-based technologies, it is becoming possible to detect evidence of many infections, such as chlamydia, gonorrhoea, Trichomonas vaginalis, and HSV-2 in a first void (i.e. the first 10–15 ml) urine sample using a single multiplex assay.[7] In addition, HIV antibodies can be detected in urine, albeit with slightly lower sensitivity than in blood.[8] Levels of β-HCG in urine can also be used to detect evidence of pregnancy. Urine is thus a useful specimen, as many of the relevant outcomes can be detected using a single specimen, and collection is not invasive. However, in some communities people may be reluctant to provide urine because of local beliefs. For example, some communities in Zimbabwe believe that a person can be bewitched by someone who has their urine.

It is likely that the number of available tests will increase considerably over the next few years. For example, the range of infections that can be reliably detected using rapid point of care technology will increase. Rapid tests have the advantage of being feasible to conduct in the field, often by non-laboratory personnel, and not requiring sophisticated laboratory facilities. Additionally, it is becoming possible to detect antibodies to an increasing number of infections in saliva and urine. Furthermore, as mentioned previously, strategies for detecting recent sero conversion to HIV have already been developed, and this technique is likely to be extended to other infections, such as HSV-2, in the near future.

Predictive value of the assay

The predictive value of a test is the probability of it being truly positive given a positive test result, or truly negative given a negative test result. The positive and negative predictive value of an assay varies according to the prevalence of the marker within a population. An infection detected in a population in which the prevalence of that infection is low is more likely to be falsely positive than it will be in a population with high prevalence. This has important implications if the biological marker is being used as a gold standard against which, for example, behavioural data are being compared.

Primary route of infection acquisition

For some infections, the primary route of acquisition/transmission varies between populations. For example, in sub-Saharan Africa, HIV is largely sexually transmitted, whereas in parts of Asia and Eastern Europe it is also commonly transmitted through injecting drug use. By contrast, HSV-2, Neisseria gonorrhoea, and Chlamydia trachomatis are mostly transmitted sexually in all populations.

Association between infection and behaviour

Direct and linear relationships between biological markers and risk behaviours are rare. Many factors determine whether risk behaviours can be detected by biological measures, such as the nature and consistency of a practice, the characteristics and transmissability of the STI, and sexual mixing patterns and STI prevalence within a given population.

Additionally, the relationship between incident STIs and incident HIV is complex.[9] Most STIs, including HIV-1, can be transmitted by anal, vaginal, and oral intercourse, each with different degrees of efficiency. This may make interpretation of biological markers problematic. For example, the presence of urethral gonorrhoea in a gay man could either indicate unprotected insertive oral sex with a man who has pharyngeal gonorrhoea or unprotected insertive anal intercourse with a man with rectal gonorrhoea. The risk of acquisition of HIV is markedly different for the two activities. It would therefore be unwise to use the presence or absence of urethral gonorrhoea as a proxy for HIV risk behaviour, although it may be a useful indicator of broader sexual risk-taking.

Little is known about whether susceptibility to infection remains the same over time. It is not known, for example, whether an individual becomes less susceptible to genital chlamydial infection with repeated infection, as occurs for trachoma (i.e. occular chlamydial infection).[10] Acquired immunity could, in part, explain the very high rates of infection among adolescent girls relative to older women. If this is the case, then young study participants may acquire infection with less-risky behaviour than older study participants, again making interpretation of the results difficult.

Acceptability and feasibility

The feasibility and acceptability of sample collection in various settings will clearly have implications for which outcome measures can be used. The potential benefits of extensive biological testing need to be set against the costs. Collecting, processing and testing large numbers of biological specimens is expensive and logistically complicated. Moreover, in some, but not all, settings, it may have a deleterious effect on response and follow-up rates.

Ethics of using biological outcome measures

Detecting infection among individuals taking part in a study clearly confers a responsibility on study investigators at least to provide treatment at the level of the local standard of care for those individuals found to be infected. In some situations, it may be desirable to unlink the biological results from other identifying information, in order to maximize response rates. The unlinking makes it impossible to link the specimen to the person who provided it. For example, individuals may be more willing to participate in an anonymous, unlinked HIV-testing study than in one that is merely confidential. In this situation, voluntary HIV counselling and testing should be made available to those participants who desire it outside of the study, with ongoing medical support provided for individuals found to be infected.

Increasingly, it is seen as ethically unacceptable to test samples for an infection or condition for which consent was not specifically sought at the time of the original study. This could result in valuable collections of stored samples and behavioural data being unusable at some point in the future, in the event of a novel and possibly as yet unenvisioned assay becoming available. When obtaining written consent from trial participants, researchers may thus wish to ask for permission to test stored samples in an unlinked manner, for assays other than those specifically stated.

Behavioural outcome measures

In a population with low prevalence of STI, a very large trial will be needed to demonstrate a significant reduction in STI following intervention. In such cases, behavioural or psychological variables can play an important role in assessing the efficacy and effectiveness of an intervention. In addition, even where biological measures are feasible and appropriate, behavioural and cognitive measures can help explain the biological impact of an intervention (i.e. how and why specific intervention components were or were not effective, or how and why specific behaviours did or did not change).

Behavioural research focusing on health-seeking practices, sexual activities, and other risk behaviours can employ both quantitative and qualitative data, and ideally involve a combination of both.[11,12] For example, in-depth qualitative research can be invaluable in determining appropriate language for quantitative survey instruments. In turn, quantitative research can provide a relatively representative overview of health-seeking or sexual practices within a cohort. Whether quantitative or qualitative data are employed, sexual behaviours can be measured by a number of different methods.[13] Self-reported behaviour can be measured using, for example, a self-completion questionnaire or a face-to-face interview. Behaviour can even be externally evaluated (i.e. directly observed using ethnographic research or simulated clients). Each of these methods will be discussed in the next section.

Self-reported behaviour

In a face-to-face interview, an interviewer directly asks questions of one or more individuals, while, in a self-completion questionnaire, participants answer questions on paper or on a computer, entirely or largely without assistance from an interviewer. Face-to-face interviews generally have greater response rates and less missing data than self-completion questionnaires.[14] They can offer more clarity and be easier to use for subjects with low literacy levels, which makes this a particularly valuable method in a developing country context. Face-to-face interviews carried out with more than one individual, as in focus group discussions (FGD), may be an economical way of learning the views of more than one person at a time, while allowing participants to engage and explore ideas amongst themselves, rather than simply responding to questions posed by an interviewer.

However, self-completion questionnaire surveys of large populations are likely to be much less costly than surveys employing face-to-face interviews. Furthermore, self-completion questionnaires may be modified for use with semi-literate or illiterate participants. A self-completion questionnaire may make use of icons rather than words, and an interviewer may read all questions aloud, but enable participants to answer them independently. Given the sensitive nature of sexual behaviour and related health-seeking practices, confidentiality is likely to be an important issue for participants, and may make face-to-face interventions, and especially focus groups, an unattractive prospect. Self-completion questionnaires may give participants a greater sense of confidentiality, whilst also reducing interviewer bias and cost.

Audio computer-assisted self-interviewing (ACASI), in which a participant completes a questionnaire on computer, may combine the best attributes of both traditional self-completion questionnaires and face-to-face interviews. Specifically, questions may be tailored to each individual and explanations provided upon request in multiple languages, while interviewer bias is reduced and completion rates increased. ACASI is still a fairly new and relatively untested method for participants with low literacy levels. However, it is hoped that it can be made accessible to such participants through the use of images, colours, numbers and an audio component.

However, whatever method is used, self-reported behaviour related to sexual health may be inaccurate for a number of reasons. For example, a participant may have poor recall, may misinterpret the question, and/or may intentionally provide inaccurate information. These will be discussed in some detail in the following section.

Social desirability bias

Because of the sensitive nature of sexual behaviour and related health-seeking practices, the potential for a participant to misreport behaviour can be high, especially if he or she believes that behaviour to be particularly socially desirable or undesirable.[15] This self-presentational bias may be even more likely if the participant has participated in an intervention in which targeted behaviours are clearly identified. Generally, researchers thus assume that socially stigmatized and/or undesirable behaviours are more likely to be under-reported than over-reported, so that higher reporting of such activities is interpreted as more valid. This may be true for sexual behaviour in general, as well as for particularly behaviours, such as homosexuality, which are heavily stigmatized in many cultures. However, assumptions about what is socially desirable can be problematic. Something that may be considered undesirable within one culture or sub-culture may be perceived as highly desirable in another. For example, machismo in some cultures may lead young men to embellish their sexual experience, wishing to demonstrate their developing sexual prowess or attractiveness, while patriarchal cultures may encourage young women to under-report their sexual experience, out of concern for their social reputation.

Interviewer characteristics such as race, class, sex, age, status, or accent all may also contribute to social desirability bias. For example, in a multiple-study, longitudinal research project in rural Uganda, Huygens et al.[16] found that female informants were more willing to provide information on rape and on sex during menstruation if they were interviewed by women rather than men. In another example,[17] some researchers found that interviewers who are uncomfortable with certain sexual behaviours may, when asking questions about those activities, provide participants with cues that suggest that the interviewer holds negative opinions about them, thereby encouraging under-reporting.

Across most self-reported sexual behaviour research methods, there are a number of components that are believed to promote honesty, and thus data validity. These include a non-judgemental approach, a permissive interview style, an appropriate setting, the use of neutral questions, and assurances of confidentiality or anonymity. Many studies also set out to explain the research, and its broader implications, to the participants, in order to encourage the participant to see the research as credible. Researchers also may attempt to assess the validity of sensitive self-reported behaviour by using internal or external consistency checks, such as comparing an individual's responses to the same or similar questions within a research instrument, or to externally measured data. For example, in a study in school children in rural Zimbabwe, only 13 per cent (95% CI 4–27) of those shown to be infected with HIV and/or another STI reported ever having sexual intercourse.[53]

Recall bias

Even if a participant intends to answer questions honestly, he or she may misunderstand a question or have poor recall, and thus report information incorrectly. Studies of memory have generally found that unless an experience was somehow particularly significant (e.g. a first sexual experience), the longer the period of time since an event occurred, the poorer the recall.[18,19] Similarly, when asked to recall event frequency, the greater the frequency of an event, the less accurate the recall.[20] For example, participants with a large number of lifetime sexual partners tend to estimate the total number in round numbers, whereas participants with few such partners provide more accurate estimates.[18] In another example, participants with infrequent unprotected sex acts demonstrate a greater reporting accuracy for unprotected acts compared with protected acts.[21] Finally, the pattern of sexual activity itself may affect recall. For example, a monogamous person with a routine pattern of sexual activity may produce highly reliable behavioural estimates, while people with more complex patterns across time and with several partners may have more difficulty.

Some ways in which researchers attempt to encourage the quality of recall include establishing a sequential stream of events over time, using a two-dimensional life history calendar grid in which concurrent events can be considered simultaneously, and/or focusing on 'landmark' events around which other events can be chronologically structured.

Interpretation of questions and answers

Self-reported information may also be inaccurate if the language used in the research instrument is not appropriate to the target community. This can be particularly challenging for research on behaviour related to sexual health. Terms that may be clear and acceptable to one individual may be ambiguous and/or offensive to another. For example, while pre-testing instruments for a UK national sexual behaviour survey in the late 1980s, Wellings et al.[11] learned that some participants found vernacular terms offensive, while some did not understand formal terms, and others made widely variable interpretations of specific terms such as 'sexual partners' or 'having sex'. Similarly, when working in rural Uganda, Hugyens et al. found that interviewers and participants sometimes conceptualized terms such as 'abstinence', 'casual partner', 'steady partner', and 'rape' quite differently.[16] Other researchers have voiced similar concerns about participant's understanding of the medical terminology used in many surveys. For example, in a study of high-risk US adolescents, Clark et al.[22] found that, comparing reported STIs and pregnancies with medical records, substantial under-reporting may have resulted from limited participant understanding of the survey terminology or of their STI diagnosis.

Approaches that may improve sexual behaviour question comprehension include: having the interviewer provide both formal and slang terms; verbally describing the sexual activity in question; and/or showing participants drawings or pictures of the behaviour in question. Where questionnaire translation is required, repeated back-translation, pilot-testing, and editing for conceptual equivalence can help minimize biases produced by lack of clarity.

Externally-evaluated behaviour

Given the many reasons why self-reported behaviour may be inaccurate, corroboration or supplementation with externally-reported or observational methods can be an important means of collecting valid data on sexual health-related behaviour.

Participant observation

In participant observation, for example, researchers may live and work among participants, sharing in daily activities while independently documenting informal interviews and observations related to sexual health. Given the private nature of sexual behaviour, participant observation in a literal sense has rarely been used to research this topic. However, it may be possible to observe some relevant behaviours, such as sexual negotiation or health-seeking practices. For example, in a study in rural Ghana, Bleek,[23] learned a great deal about abortion by what he observed before and after abortion procedures, although he himself never actually saw one. However, weaknesses of participant observation can include a limited ability to direct the focus of the research and problems of representativeness.

Simulated clients

This method aims to assess one aspect of sexual health-related behaviour, namely the practice of health care workers. In the simulated client method, research assistants, who have fictitious case scenarios, stable conditions, or a genuine interest in the services, visit providers and request their assistance using standardized scenarios. During the visit, providers are not aware that those particular clients are engaged in research. However, for ethical reasons they should have been previously informed that such research may be conducted with them during a broad time period. The simulated clients later report the events of the visit to a research supervisor and the data are analysed. Like participant observation, the simulated client method provides data that would be difficult or impossible to obtain through other research methods. Rather than assessing knowledge, competence or performance, which can all be assessed through other means, the simulated client method provides an opportunity to record unselfconscious, actual practice, from the point of view of a client in a first-hand, standardized account. It thus provides a very important complement to self-reported practices. However, limitations of simulated client research include concerns about representativeness, difficulty in generalizing a standardized scenario to other kinds of health problems, and minimal insight into the characteristics, technical understanding, opinions, and motivations of the providers or actual users.

Other methods of external evaluation of outcomes

Other methods to assess behaviour externally can be used to determine intervention effectiveness. For example, many countries maintain registers of abortion, births or cancer statistics. These data are usually kept confidential, but it still may be possible for researchers to glean useful, unlinked information from such registries. For example, researchers can give the guardians of the register a file containing identifying information on study participants, according to intervention or comparison group. The registries are then able to provide statistics on the number of abortions, births, or cervical cancers that occurred in each arm of the trial. This serves as a useful means of validating self-reports, and in the case of national registers with high rates of registration, may have few problems of loss to follow up, providing participants use the same identifying information for both the study and the register. For example, in a randomized trial of school-based sex education in the UK, the incidence of abortion will be determined through linkage of all female participants to national abortion data that are known to be very complete.

Condom sales and/or distribution figures can also be used to corroborate self-reports of condom use at a population level. Alternatively, several studies have actually ascertained condom use by collecting used condoms from outdoor sex venues, or by looking for direct evidence of condom use in vacated hotel rooms.[24] The possibility that such measures reflect a particular mode of disposal, rather than use, of condoms should however be borne in mind.

Psychological outcome measures

In addition to biological or behavioural outcome measures, many researchers select cognitive and other psychological outcome measures that are believed to be antecedents or determinants of risk reduction. Cognitions associated with reduced risk can be as simple as basic knowledge about HIV/AIDS, or as complex as an individual's perceptions of social norms and susceptibility to risk, or sense of self-efficacy.[25] These individual outcome measures can be grouped under inter-related categories, such as attitudes and beliefs (e.g. perceived barriers to, attractiveness of, and consequences of condom use) or personality variables (e.g. impulsivity or risk-taking tendency).[26]

As with selection of biological or behavioural outcome measures, any cognitive or psychological outcome measures should be identified early in a trial, as they will influence trial design. Relevant psychological outcomes are identified in various psychological models of behaviour (see Chapter 4). These aim to enable the nature of the health issue to be understood, the needs and motivations of the target population to be specified, and the appropriate context of the intervention to be considered. However, reviews of sexual behaviour interventions have found that most of these are, in fact, based on an informal blend of common sense and practical experience, rather than explicit theory. Reviewers conclude that such interventions and their evaluation could be improved with underpinning by one or more theories.[27–29] Some of the more influential theories for sexual behaviour interventions and research have been the Health Belief Model, the Theory of Planned Behaviour, the AIDS Risk Reduction Model (ARRM) and Social Learning Theory. (See Chapter 4)

Psychological outcome measures have many of the same advantages and limitations as behavioural measures. Cognitive data can be collected quantitatively, for representativeness, or qualitatively, for in-depth understanding. They can be self-reported or externally measured. They may provide a relatively simple means of assessing intervention impact, and importantly, can provide valuable insight into the subtle and complex process of an intervention, and the relative effectiveness of its different components.

However, like behavioural variables, self-reported cognitive outcome measures may be subject to social desirability or self-presentational bias, particularly in an intervention context where participants are aware of the cognitions and behaviours targeted by the intervention. At best, it may be possible to identify and reduce such bias through triangulation of methods.

Conclusions

The choice of outcome measures used to assess intervention effectiveness will depend on logistical as well as scientific factors. Biological outcome measures have several advantages over behavioural and cognitive measures. Biological measures are not prone to reporting bias, and thus may provide more valid data than self-reported measures. In addition, interventions that have been shown to reduce rates of STIs or unintended pregnancy are likely to carry more weight with policy-makers than those that have only been shown to change sexual behaviour or cognitions.

However, biological measures are not necessarily a gold standard, as they may be prone to other kinds of error, such as false positive or negative results, as well as limited and complex association between outcomes and behaviours. In many contexts, it may be neither feasible nor affordable to collect biological specimens. Finally, while biological outcome measures alone may demonstrate that an intervention has had the desired impact, they provide little insight into the effectiveness of different intervention components or the effect of the intervention on behavioural and psychological factors.

The aim of the intervention, the context in which it is being conducted, and the available facilities and resources will all influence the decision about which outcome measures to choose. It is important that the limitations of the various measures are taken into account when planning the study, and that attempts are made to minimize these. Triangulating complementary outcome measures will likely provide the most useful information on the effectiveness of the intervention, and may also help to explain how that effect, or lack of effect, was brought about.

References

1. Peterman, T.A., Lin, L.S., Newman, D.R., *et al.* (2000) Does measured behaviour reflect STD risk? *Sex Transm Dis*, **27**, 446–51.

2. Obasi, A., Mosha, F., Quigley, M., *et al.* (1999) Antibody to herpes simplex virus type 2 as a marker of sexual risk behaviour in rural Tanzania. *J Infect Dis*, **179**, 16–24.

3. McFarland, W., Lovemore, G., Bassett, M.T., *et al.* (1999) Prevalence and incidence of herpes simplex virus type 2 infection among male Zimbabwean factory workers. *J Infect Dis*, **180**, 1459–65.

4. Zenilman, J., Rogers, S.M., Forel, N.C., *et al.* (2001) Detecting sperm DNA in vaginal swabs by PCR: a new bio-marker to validate recent sexual behaviour and condom use. *Int J STD AIDS*, **12**(suppl. 2), 60.

5. Janssen, R.S., Statten, G.A., Stramer, S.L., *et al.* (1998) New testing strategy to detect early HIV-1 infection for use in incidence estimates and for clinical and prevention purposes. *JAMA*, **280**, 42–48.

6. Tabrizi, S.N., Fairley, C.K., Chen, S., *et al.* (2000) Evaluation of patient-administered tampon specimens for Chlamydia trachomatis and Neisseria gonorrhoeae. *Sex Transm Dis*, **27**, 133–37.

7. Tabrizi, S.N., Skov, S., Chandeying, V., Norpech, J., and Garland, S.M. (2000) Prevalence of sexually transmitted infections among clients of female commercial sex workers in Thailand. *Sex Transm Dis*, **24**, 358–61.

8. Mortimer, P.P. and Parry, J.V. (1995) Non-invasive virological diagnosis: are saliva and urine specimens adequate for blood. *Rev Med Virol*, **1**, 73–8.

9. Fishbein, M. and Jarvis, B. (2000) Failure to find a behavioral surrogate for STD incidence—what does it really mean? *Sex Transm Dis*, **27**, 452–5.

10. Bailey, R., Duong, T., Carpenter, B., Norpech, J., and Garland, S.M. (1999) The duration of human ocular chlamydial infection is age dependent. *Epidemiol Infect*, **123**, 479–86.

11. Wellings, K., Field, J., Wadsworth, J., Johnson, A.M., Anderson, R.M., and Bradshaw, S. (1990) Sexual lifestyles under scrutiny. *Nature*, **348**, 276–8.

12. Ankrah, E.M. (1989) AIDS: methodological problems in studying its prevention and spread. *Soc Sci Med*, **29**, 265–76.

13. Fenton, K.A., Johnson, A.M., McManus, S., and Erens, B. (2001) Measuring sexual behaviour: methodological challenges in survey research. *Sex Transm Infect*, 77, 84–92.

14. Hingson, R. and Strunin, L. (1993) Validity, reliability, and generalizability in studies of AIDS knowledge, attitudes and behavioral risks based on subject self-report. *Am J Prev Med*, 9, 62–4.

15. Copas, A.J., Wellings, K., Erens, B., *et al.* (2002) The accuracy of reported sensitive sexual behaviour in Britain: exploring the extent of change 1990–2000. *Sex Transm Infect*, 78, 26–30.

16. Huygens, P., Kajura, E., Seeley, J., Johnson, A.M., Anderson, R.M., and Bradshaw, S. (1996) Rethinking methods for the study of sexual behaviour. *Soc Sci Med*, 42, 221–31.

17. Catania, J.A., Turner, H., and Pierce, R., *et al.* (1993) Response bias in surveys of AIDS-related sexual behavior. In: Ostrow, D.G. and Kessler, R.C. (eds) *Methodological Issues in AIDS Behavioral Research*. Plenum Press, New York.

18. Morris, M. (1993) Telling tails explain the discrepancy in sexual partner reports. *Nature*, 365, 437–40.

19. Kauth, M.R., St Lawrence, J.S., and Kelly, J.A. (1991) Reliability of retrospective assessments of sexual HIV risk behavior: a comparison of biweekly, three-month, and twelve-month self-reports. *AIDS Educ Prev*, 3, 207–14.

20. Catania, J.A., Gibson, D.R., Chitwood, D.D., and Coates, T.J. (1990) Methodological problems in AIDS behavioral research: influences on measurement error and participation bias in studies of sexual behaviour. *Psychol Bull*, 108, 339–62.

21. McFarlane, M. and St. Lawrence, J.S. (1999) Adolescents' recall of sexual behavior: consistency of self-report and effect of variations in recall duration. *J Adolesc Health*, 25, 199–206.

22. Clark, L.R., Brasseux, C., and Richmond, D. (1997) Are adolescents accurate in self-report of frequencies of sexually transmitted diseases and pregnancies? *J Adolesc Health*, 21, 91–6.

23. Bleek, W. (1987) Lying informants: a fieldwork experience from Ghana. *Popul Dev Rev* 13, 314–22.

24. Egger, M., Pauw, J., Lopatatzidis, A., Medrano, D., Paccaud, F., and Davey Smith, G. (2000) Promotion of condom use in a high-risk setting in Nicaragua: a randomized controlled trial. *Lancet*, 355, 2101–5.

25. O'Leary, A., Goodhart, F., Jemmott, L., and Boccher-Lattimore, D. (1992) Predictors of safer sex on the college campus: a social cognitive theory analysis. *J Am Coll Health*, 40, 254–63.

26. Sheeran, P., Abraham, C., and Orbel, S. (1999) Psychosocial correlates of heterosexual condom use: a meta-analysis. *Psychol Bull*, 125, 90–132.

27. Kirby, D., Short, L., Collins, J., *et al.* (1994) School-based programmes to decrease sexual risk behaviours: a review of effectiveness. *Public Health Rep*, 109, 339–60.

28. Wight, D., Abraham, C., and Scott, S. (1998) Towards a psycho-social theoretical framework for sexual health promotion. *Health Educ Res*, 13(3), 317–30.

29. Stuart-Smith, S. (1996) Teenage sex: cognitive immaturity increases the risks. *Br Med J*, 312, 390–1.

30. WHO. (2001) Guidelines for Using HIV Testing Technologies in Surveillance: Selection, Evaluation and Implementation. *WHO/UNAIDS Publication*: WHO/CDS/EDC/2001.16.

31. Ashley, R.L. (2001) Sorting out the new HSV type specific antibody tests. *Sex Transm Infect*, **77**, 232–7.

32. Mason, P.R., Gregson, S., Gwanzura, L., Cappuccinelli, P., Rapelli, P., and Fiori, P.L. (2001) Enzyme immunoassay for urogenital trichomoniasis as a marker of unsafe sexual behaviour. *Epidemiol Infect*, **126**, 103–9.

33. Newhall, W.J., Johnson, R.E., DeLisle, S., *et al.* (1999) Head-to-head evaluation of five chlamydia tests relative to a quality-assured culture standard. *J Clin Microbiol*, **37**, 681–5.

34. Sparling, P.F. (1999) The biology of Neisseria gonorrhoeae. In: Holmes, K.K., Sparling, P.F., Mardh, P.A., *et al.* (eds) *Sexually Transmitted Diseases*. McGraw- Hill, New York, pp. 433–49.

35. Desjardins, M., Thompson, C.E., Filion, L.G., *et al.* (1992) Standardization of enzyme immunoassay for human antibdoy to Haemophilus ducreyi. *J Clin Microbiol*, **30**, 2019–24.

36. Wagner, H.U., Van Dyck, E., Roggen E., *et al.* (1994) Seroprevalence and incidence of sexually transmitted diseases in a rural Ugandan population. *Int J STD AIDS*, **5**, 332–7.

37. Freinkel, A., Dangor, Y., Koornof, H., and Ballard, R. (1992) A serological test for granuloma inguinale. *Genitourin Med*, **68**, 269–72.

38. Egglestone, S.I. and Turner, A.L.J. (2000) Serological diagnosis of syphilis. *Community Dis Public Health*, **3**, 158–62.

39. Young, H. (2000) Guidelines for serological testing of syphilis. *Sex Transm Infect*, **76**, 403–5.

40. UNAIDS and WHO. (1998) *Laboratory Requirements for the Safe and Effective Use of Antiretrovirals*.

41. Black, C.M. (2002) Current methods of laboratory diagnosis of *Chlamydia trachomatis* Infections. *Clin Microbiol Rev*, **10**, 160–84.

42. Peeling, R.W., Toye, B., Jessamine, P., and Gemmill, I. (1998) Pooling of urine specimens for PCR testing: a cost saving strategy for Chlamydia trachomatis control programmes. *Sex Transm Infect*, **74**, 66–70.

43. Van der Pol, B., Quinn, T.C., Gaydos, C.A., *et al.* (2000) Multicenter evaluation of the AMPLICOR and automated COBAS AMPLICOR CT/NG tests for detection of Chlamydia trachomatis. *J Clin Microbiol*, **38**, 1105–12.

44. Van der Pol, B., Martin, D.H., Schachter, J., *et al.* (2001) Enhancing the specificity of the COBAS AMPLICOR CT/NG test for Neisseria gonorrhoeae by retesting specimens with equivocal results. *J Clin Microbiol*, **39**, 3092–8.

45. Jephcott, A. (1997) Microbiological diagnosis of gonorrhoea. *Genitourin Med*, **73**, 245–52.

46. Patel, S.R., Wiese, W., Patel, S.C., Ohl, C., Byrd, J.C., and Estrada, C.A. (2000) Systematic review of diagnostic tests for vaginal trichomoniasis. *Infect Dis Obstet Gynecol*, **8**, 248–57.

47. Rompalo, A.M., Gaydos, C.A., Shah, N., *et al.* (2001) Evaluation of use of a single intravaginal swab to detect multiple sexually transmitted infections in active-duty military women. *Clin Infect Dis*, **33**, 1455–61.

48. Chernesky, M.A. (1999) Nucleic acid tests for the diagnosis of sexually transmitted diseases. *FEMS Immunol Med Microbiol*, **24**, 437–46.

49. Clark, A.M., Steece, R., Crouse, K., *et al.* (2001) Multisite pooling study using ligase chain reaction in screening for genital Chlamydia trachomatis infections. *Sex Transm Dis*, **28**, 565–8.

50. Van Dyck, E., Ieven, M., Pattyn, S., Van Damme, L., and Laga, M. (2001) Detection of Chlamydia trachomatis and Neisseria gonorrhoeae by enzyme immunoassay, culture, and three nucleic acid amplification tests. *J Clin Microbiol*, **39**, 1751–6.

51. Safrin, S., Shaw, H., Bolan, G., Cuan, J., and Chiang, C.S. (1997) Comparison of virus culture and the polymerase chain reaction for diagnosis of mucocutaneous herpes simplex virus infection. *Sex Transm Dis*, **24**, 176–80.

52. Orle, K.A., Gates, C.A., Martin, D.H., and Boyde, B.A. (1996) Simultaneous PCR detection of Haemophilis ducrei, Trepanoma pallidum and herpes simplex type 1 and 2 from genital ulcers. *J Clin Microbiol*, **34**, 49–54.

53. Cowan, F.N., Langhaug, L.F., Mashungupa, GP., Nyamurera, T., Hargrove, J., Jaffar, S., Peeling, R.N., Brown, D.N.G., Power, R., Stephenson, J.M., Bassett, M.T., and Hayes, R.J. for the Dzive Shiri Project. (2002) School based HIV prevention in Zimbabwe: feasibility and acceptability of evaluation trials using biological outcomes. *AIDS*, **16**, 1673–8.

Chapter 9

Developing and validating complex behavioural outcome measures

Rochelle N. Shain, Sondra Perdue, Jeanna M. Piper, Alan E.C. Holden, Jane Champion, and Edward R. Newton

Introduction

Interventions developed to reduce the risk of infection with sexually transmitted infections (STIs) have typically focused on changes in discrete behaviours. However, simple behaviours alone may not be directly related to risk of infection. The purpose of this chapter is to examine the types of behavioural measures commonly used, and to explore the development of complex measures. The utility of each will be considered with reference to data from randomized controlled trials (RCTs) that have utilized both biological and behavioural measures.

Many STI/HIV risk-reduction interventions, tested in RCTs, have successfully changed aspects of condom-use behaviour in one or both genders.[1–8] Change in partner-related behaviours, such as partner number and partner type, have been reported less frequently, and have met with limited success.[1,2,6] Few RCTs have used infection as an outcome measure,[1–4, 8–10] and only two successfully reduced the rate of new infections.[1,2,11] Data from both of these trials have been used to examine the relationship between infection and behaviour measured by responses to interview questions.[1,12–16] This type of analysis can provide insight into which behaviours were modified by the intervention, and the extent to which these changes influenced infection rates. Specifically, Project RESPECT found minimal association between infection and behavioural measures,[16] whereas Project SAFE,[1,12–14] using more comprehensive measures incorporating context, found more significant relationships.

It is important to gain insight into the complex relationship between infection and behaviour to learn: (a) which behaviours or combinations of behaviours must be changed in order to reduce the rate of new infection; and (b) meaningful ways to measure sexual behaviours so that they reflect actual likelihood of infection. This is especially important because many STI/HIV prevention studies rely on behavioural outcomes, primarily those pertaining to condom use, to evaluate intervention efficacy. The purpose of this chapter is to examine the relationship between infection and: (a) simple and complex measures of commonly used behavioural variables; (b) less commonly used behavioural measures; and (c) complex measures, considered simultaneously. Discussion relies primarily on data from Project SAFE,[1,12,14] but also refers to results from Project RESPECT.[2,16,17] This chapter suggests that links between measured behaviours and biology are clarified when behaviours are purpose-fully examined as more holistic entities and considered jointly.[12,14,15] The use of biological and behavioural outcomes is also discussed in Chapter 8.

Project SAFE characteristics

This behavioural risk-reduction intervention was designed for Mexican- and African-American women and evaluated in an RCT, stratified by ethnicity. All 617 participants had a non-viral STI at baseline. They were screened and treated for STIs, and interviewed at baseline, and at six- and twelve-month follow-ups. Visits included physical examinations and laboratory tests. Participants could also return to the research clinic between scheduled visits if they experienced particular problems. The follow-up rate at twelve-months was 89 per cent, with a sample of 549. The biologic outcome measure was infection with gonorrhea and/or chlamydia. Study procedures are described in greater detail in the original publication.[1]

Data presented here are based on the subset of 477 women with complete data from both follow-up visits. Unless otherwise indicated, results are from the cumulative follow-up period zero-to-twelve months and reflect worst-case values; women were assigned to the lower-risk category cumulatively only if they were low-risk in that measure at both six- and twelve-months. Data on condom-use measures reflect behaviour during the last three months of the zero-to-six or six-to-twelve month interval, or in the case of the cumulative measure, both three-month intervals. Baseline sample characteristics and infection rates for the 477 women are similar to those previously described for the entire follow-up sample.[1,14] A more complete analysis of behavioural and biological data can be found elsewhere.[14]

Commonly used measures of sexual behaviour

Partner number and type

Simple constructs

Few studies refer to the number and type of partner to explain STI rate reduc-tions.[1,13,16] Results reported from Project RESPECT indicate that having three or more partners in a six-month interval was associated with infection (adjusted odds ratio = 1.9)[16]. In Project SAFE, various partner-number cut-offs were associated with infection. During the twelve-month study period, participants with one or no partner had an infection rate of 14.9 per cent, compared with 32.6 per cent for those with two or more partners ($p < 0.001$).[1] Women with three or more partners had an infection rate of 37.9 per cent, compared with 17.5 per cent ($p < 0.001$) for those with two or fewer partners.

Project RESPECT interventions focused on consistent condom use.[2] However, data were collected on partner type (main vs occasional partners), and used as a stratification variable for the number of unprotected acts,[16] discussed in the condom-use section below. Project SAFE focused on a number of issues, including partner relationships. Consequently, a great deal of attention was given to partner measurements. One potential source of measurement error can be the varying definitions given to the word 'steady' by different participants.[14] To minimize this error, Project SAFE researchers classified relationships reported to be steady 'all or most of the time' as steady. 'Off-and-on' steady relationships and any type of steady relationship reported by married women living apart from their spouses because of marital difficulties were classified as casual. This category also included occasional partners, those a woman had just met, someone who provides drugs, etc. It seemed, from initial research with similar populations, that such relationships were often high risk: partners frequently had sex with others during the 'off' periods and during separation. Participants often continued to have occasional sex with these partners, despite their separated status.

The results support this definition. During Project SAFE's twelve-month follow-up period, 344 women reported that they had steady partners exclusively; their infection rate was 15.4 per cent. The 104 women whose relationships were steady 'off and on' (i.e. casual according to the definition used), had a rate of 23.1 per cent, compared with 12.1 per cent for the 240 participants whose relationships were steady all or most of the time.

Composite constructs

The number of partners, along with the nature of these relationships, also affects infection rates. Women with one 'steady' (our definition) partner had an infection rate of 11.6 per cent, vs 18.9 per cent for those with two or more steady partners. Among women with any 'casual' partners, infection rates were 24.2 per cent for women with one partner, and 39.7 per cent for women with two or more partners. Perceived partner fidelity also affected the likelihood of infection. To increase precision, a 'mutual monogamy' variable was created, conceptualized to include type of relationship, partner number, and fidelity.[14] The 203 women who had one steady, monogamous sex partner, or no sex during follow-up ($n = 15$) had an infection rate of 8.4 per cent compared with 31.4 per cent for everyone else ($n = 274$), translating into a risk ratio of 3.7. These refinements provided a more complete characterization of the relationship, and therefore the measure was more significantly related to infection.

Condom-use

Simple constructs

Many RCTs rely on condom-use measures to assess efficacy, because condoms can prevent transmission of some STIs, including HIV.[18] It is also relatively simple to focus on changing one aspect of sexual behaviour. Condom-use measures have included proportion of acts protected, mean number of unprotected acts, 100 per cent condom use, and no unprotected acts. The first of these is rightly noted to be very limited, because it does not consider the number of total acts; for example, 50 per cent use could mean one, or more than a hundred, unprotected acts.[19,20]

In the few instances in which infection and behavioural data are simultaneously available, it has become increasingly clear that commonly employed condom-use measures alone are not reliable predictors of disease acquisition. For example, in a Baltimore clinic, men using condoms 'all the time' were as likely to be infected as those who never used them, or who sometimes used them.[21] Re-examination of these data found no support for risk of infection varying according to level of use. The authors suggested that these anomalous results were due to systematic group differences in reporting errors, and in risk of exposure to an STI.[22] Data from Project RESPECT showed that both of the counseling intervention arms were associated with some behavioural change at follow-up. Increases in 'any condom use' and 'no unprotected vaginal sex' persisted until six months, whereas group differences in 'condom used at last sex', 'one or fewer sex partners', 'no casual partners', and 'no new partners' were found only at the three-month visit.[2] More importantly, changes in the number of unprotected acts, or the percentage of sexual acts without a condom, even after controlling for sex with a new partner, were not related to infection.[17]

Data from Project SAFE yielded similar results. Of the 462 women who had sex during the twelve-month follow-up period, 80 used condoms 'most or all of the time,' regarded as 75 per cent of the time. Their infection rate was 21.3 per cent, compared with 22.5 per cent for those who did not use condoms, or used them less frequently. The variable 'mean number of unprotected acts' was not associated with infection (Pearson's $r = -0.01$).[14] Only 41 women had no unprotected acts; their infection rate was 14.6 per cent compared with 22.3 per cent for everyone else ($p = 0.26$). The non-significant lower rate was due to zero infections among the 15 women with no sex. The 26 participants who used condoms all the time had an infection rate of 23.1 per cent, compared with 22.2 per cent for the remaining participants. Hence, these simple predictors were not appropriate indicators of infection in this study.

Although 26 women is a small sub-set, it is instructive to examine the behaviour of the three infected women who reported 100 per cent condom use. They had infections only during the first six-month interval; two at problem visits, and one at the six-month screen. They probably provided accurate reports about condom use, which referred only to the last three months of that interval. However, their responses to another question indicated that none of the three women used condoms initially following enrollment. All reported they had unprotected sex with partners for whom they could not be sure of complete treatment following the baseline infection. Other researchers[2,3,16] have also utilized a recall period of the last three months because it covers a sufficiently long period of time to be representative, but does not present a large recall burden. However, in the absence of detailed data from other questions, it was not possible to know what had actually happened. Even had behaviour been measured every three months and achieved complete ascertainment, assessment of the effect of 100 per cent condom use would have been limited by the small number of participants who practised it.

A more useful way of conceptualizing unprotected acts is a specific cut-off point during a given interval of time.[1] In project SAFE, fewer than five unprotected acts during two three-month periods more accurately discriminated the infected from the uninfected than other condom-use measures; women with five or more acts were more than twice as likely to be infected than those with fewer unprotected acts than this.[1,14] Although fewer than five unprotected acts yielded a useful cumulative measure, it was not a significant predictor of infection at zero-to-six or six-to-twelve months: the shorter-term measures were confounded by women who had very few coital acts, all of which were unprotected sex with a casual partner (see the definition above). Over time, represented by the cumulative measure, many of these participants shifted to a higher number of unprotected acts. Of interest, in this population fewer than five unprotected acts affected the likelihood of infection only among women with riskier relationships; for example, among participants with only steady partners, infection rates were 9.5 per cent and 11.0 per cent, respectively, for women with low and high frequency of unprotected acts. On the other hand, among women with any casual partners, the infection rate was 12.7 per cent for those with fewer than five unprotected acts, compared with 38.2 per cent for those with five or more ($p < 0.001$). Project RESPECT found similar results:[16] six or more acts with an occasional partner, but not with a steady partner, was related to infection with an odds ratio of 1.9.

Composite constructs

Successful condom use depends not only on the consistency, but also correctness, of use.[12,14,23] Participants who reported breakage, slippage, or other problems such as the condom becoming dislodged inside the vagina, were classified as having problematic use. Ethnographic data indicated that, in order to retain some flesh contact, some couples only applied the condom partially, occasionally resulting in its being retained inside the vagina. Consequently, women were asked if they routinely checked that the penis was completely covered; if they did not, they too were considered to have problematic use. Of interest, a negative response to this question was more strongly related to infection than were reports of slippage and breakage. Of the 141 condom-users with problems, the 59 who did not check that the penis was covered had an infection rate of 42.4 per cent, compared with 21.7 per cent for those with other problems. Thus, the addition of this dimension of condom-use behaviour to the variable 'problematic use' improved its explanatory power.

Results indicate that, of the 331 women with any condom use during follow-up, 42.6 per cent experienced some problematic use. Their cumulative infection rate was 30.5 per cent, compared with 16.8 per cent among those without problems. Considering only those women whose cumulative acts were protected more than 75 per cent ($n = 80$), 90 per cent or more ($n = 59$), and 100 per cent ($n = 26$) of the time, respective infection rates for participants with and without problems were 24.3 per cent vs 18.6 per cent, 20.8 per cent vs 17.1 per cent, and 30.0 per cent vs 18.8 per cent. Very few participants always or almost always used condoms; whereas correct use did make a difference, it did not overcome all the problems associated with appropriately classifying individuals with regard to their condom use.

To minimize these problems, a composite variable 'unsafe sex' was created, incorporating the number of unprotected acts, problematic usage, and relationship type.[14] The variable 'unsafe sex' was designed to be partner-specific with respect to use/never-use of condoms, because of a belief that individuals choosing risky partners may compensate for this elevated risk by increasing condom use.[19,26] It was reasoned that never using condoms would be much higher risk with a casual rather than a steady partner, because it would reflect absence of any caution. These women and those who had a combination of five or more unprotected acts in three months as well as problematic use were assigned to 'unsafe sex'; all others were assigned to 'safer sex.' A participant with a casual partner would be considered high risk in the variable 'mutual monogamy', but if she used condoms with that partner, she could be considered low risk with respect to unsafe sex. Although type of relationship was included in both 'unsafe sex' and 'mutual monogamy', tests of co-linearity indicated sufficient independence.[14]

The 305 women who practised 'safer sex' had a cumulative infection rate of 13.8 per cent, whereas the 172 who experienced 'unsafe sex' had a rate 35.5 per cent (risk ratio = 2.6). Unlike five or more unprotected acts, this measure was also significantly associated with infection at both zero-to-six and six-to-twelve months.[14]

New partner

Simple constructs

Acquiring a new sex partner is assumed to increase infection risk because that individual may be an unknown entity, transmitting new infections. However, this assumption has not been adequately tested. In fact, data from Project RESPECT indicate that having a new partner is not associated with infection.[16] In Project RESPECT, partner status was determined by asking participants if a given person was a new sex partner. Project SAFE, in contrast, considered a partner 'old' only if he was listed as a sex partner in the prior six-month interval. All other men, including 'ex-steadies,' were classified 'new' because they represented potential new exposures. The 210 participants who gained a new partner anytime during follow-up had an infection rate of 31.5 per cent, compared with 16.7 per cent for those who only had 'old' partners.[14]

Composite constructs

However, this simple comparison is misleading. Of the women with 'new' partners, the 70 who waited three or more months between sex partners had an infection rate of 8.6 per cent, compared with 39.3 per cent for the 140 women who did not wait. Consequently, lack of a waiting period (i.e. either not taking three or more months to select a new partner, to have sex with him, or a combination of both) was associated with infection.[14]

The three-month waiting period may reflect selectivity and patience, or may be associated with reduced infection rates simply because waiting restricts the number of sexual partnerships that can be formed in one year. Using logistic regression analysis among the subset of 210 participants who had new partners, it was found that, by including the waiting period in the model (adjusted odds ratio=5.1), neither multiple partners (i.e. one or none vs two vs three or more), nor concurrent relationships were significantly related to infection.[14]

A new variable, 'rapid partner turnover', was created to distinguish between women who waited less than three months between sex partners from those who waited three or more months, or who did not acquire a new man. Project SAFE results indicate that the 140 women with rapid partner turnover had an infection rate of 39.3 per cent, compared with 14.2 per cent for participants with lower partner turnover (risk ratio = 2.8).[14]

Less commonly used variables

Avoiding sex with an untreated partner

Perhaps the best way to maximize re-infection risk is having unprotected sex with an untreated or incompletely treated partner. Whereas it is impossible to know the infection status of a partner unless he is tested, incomplete treatment appears to be an excellent proxy. In Project SAFE, women were asked at the six-month interview if they had sex with any partner before he completed treatment following the baseline infection. Responses were 'no,' 'yes' (with or without condoms), and 'don't know' (with or without condoms). Nurse-clinicians' notes were also used to cross-validate the responses. The 17 participants who said they did not have sex before a partner completed treatment, but who told the nurse otherwise, were considered to have had sex with an untreated man.

At six-month follow-up, 414 women had avoided unprotected sex with an untreated partner. Their infection rate was 9.4 per cent, compared with 46.0 per cent for the 63 participants who did not (risk ratio=4.9). Cumulative infection rates for these sub-sets were 16.9 per cent and 52.4 per cent, respectively (risk ratio=3.1).[12,14] A similar measure, 'avoiding *any* sex with an untreated partner,' yielded similar results.[1] Although both measures are excellent predictors of infection, having unprotected sex with an untreated partner is the better of the two, probably because it indicates exceedingly high-risk behaviour. This variable remained an indicator of infection throughout the twelve-month study period because of its strength during zero-to-six-months. In addition, some women returned to, or never left, the untreated partner. Having unprotected sex with a man thought to be untreated or incompletely treated may also reflect a propensity for risk behaviour.

Combinations

No one variable, regardless of its complexity, can provide an accurate estimate of the likelihood of infection. Sexual risk consists of various dimensions of behaviour and circumstance that are interwoven. Thus, accuracy of estimates increases when variables are combined. As noted earlier, data from Project RESPECT show that fewer than six unprotected acts in a three-month interval among women with casual partners was associated with infection, whereas it made no difference among women with only steady partners.[16] Project SAFE results were similar, using a cut-off point of fewer than five acts in two three-month intervals. This outcome makes sense, in that women with steady partners presumably have more intimate knowledge of their partners' history and current behaviour, can more accurately assess risk, and thus have a smaller likelihood of exposure to infection than women with casual partners. Using a condom in a low-risk relationship is not likely to contribute much additional prevention benefit.

Combining complex variables provides even better explanation.[12–14] In Project SAFE, the most powerful two-variable combination was mutual monogamy and avoiding unprotected sex with an untreated partner. As already noted, mutually monogamous women had an infection rate of 8.4 per cent, compared with 31.4 per cent for the non-monogamous. Participants who avoided unprotected sex with an untreated partner had an infection rate of 16.9 per cent, compared with 52.4 per cent for those who did not. When combined, the 182 mutually monogamous women who avoided such sex had an infection rate of 4.4 per cent, compared with 32.2 per cent for everyone else, who were high-risk on one or both of these behaviours. Pairing mutual monogamy with each of two other modifiable behaviours (i.e. low partner turnover or safer sex), yielded infection rates of 7.7 per cent in both cases.[14] Participants who avoided sex with an untreated partner, and had either low partner turnover or safer sex, had infection rates of 9.2 per cent, compared with 41.3 per cent and 38.1 per cent, respectively, for everyone else.

The 232 non-monogamous women who avoided sex with an untreated man had an infection rate of 26.7 per cent, whereas the 42 women with both high-risk behaviours had an infection rate of 57.1 per cent, compared with 4.4 per cent for women with neither behaviour (risk ratio = 13.0).[14] Non-monogamous women practicing safer sex had an infection rate of 23.0 per cent, similar to the rate (23.1 per cent) attained by non-monogamous women with low partner turnover. These results indicate that a mutually monogamous woman can probably avoid re-infection if she makes certain that her partner is treated or, if not, avoids unprotected sex with him (infection rate of 4.4 per cent). By definition, if a couple is mutually monogamous within the limits of measurement error, neither will become re-infected following an initial infection if both partners are adequately treated before resuming unprotected sex. However, not all women experience a mutually monogamous relationship. These women, already at higher risk, must avoid several risk behaviours in order to reduce substantively their re-infection rate. But even then, these rates do not approach those of mutually monogamous women with treated partners.[14]

Logistic regression results from a multivariate model incorporating the four risk behaviours discussed here, as well as douching after sex, demonstrated that approximately 70 per cent of re-infections may be predicted by these variables.[14] The Project SAFE intervention helped reduce infection rates because it motivated participants to: avoid unprotected sex with an untreated partner; be more cautious in partner selection (i.e. have a lower partner turnover); achieve mutual monogamy; and/or avoid very unsafe sex.[12,14]

Discussion

It has become evident that sexual behaviour change necessary to reduce STI rates is exceedingly complex, dependent on a variety of factors, including: number of partners; partner selectivity; type of relationship formed; adherence to treatment protocols on the part of both partners; and correct and consistent condom use.[1,12,14–16,19,23–26] This chapter has demonstrated that these factors do not all have to occur simultaneously for an individual to be protected. For example, mutually monogamous relationships do not require condom use if both partners are treated. In contrast, changing only one aspect of behaviour does not ensure protection from infection. For example, a woman who reduces her number of unprotected acts to only one or two in three months is nonetheless likely to be infected if those acts are with casual partners. Some behavioural changes are interdependent on others to prevent infection. Thus, a commonly used behavioural measure—number of unprotected acts—may not be a reliable predictor of infection if considered alone.

Even 100 per cent condom use, as reported in this chapter and by others,[16,21] does not necessarily discriminate between the infected and uninfected. This could be due to: faulty recall or reporting; incorrect use; lack of correspondence between the reporting periods for infection and behaviour; or other factors. In Project SAFE, one source of measurement error was that infection was screened routinely every six months, whereas the number of unprotected acts was based on the last three months of that interval. Asking women to report on behaviours in the last six months, or interviewing them every three months, may have produced different results. In a new trial,[27] respondents are being asked about their sexual behaviour in the last three and six months, in order to achieve better ascertainment. Another approach, frequent interviewing, may unduly contribute to patient burden and would make an already costly study even more expensive. Only 51 per cent of Project RESPECT participants returned for all four follow-up visits.[2] Moreover, although women in Project RESPECT were questioned every three months about their condom-use behaviour, and were screened for infection every six months, zero unprotected acts, vs everything else, was not related to infection.[16] Correctness of use was not included in this variable; perhaps it would have made a substantive difference.[24] However, it is also likely that collecting condom-use data is difficult to do without introducing a great deal of measurement error. Study participants may not recall exactly when they started to use condoms all the time, or if they stopped for any reason. Some may not realize that they, or their partners, are using condoms incorrectly. In this chapter, it has been demonstrated that several women in Project SAFE who reported consistent condom use in the last three months of each follow-up interview were, nonetheless, infected: they had had unprotected sex with an untreated partner following the baseline infection. Their responses may have been different had the time frame been the last six months. However they still may not have recalled when they began consistent condom use. The question regarding sex with an untreated partner was sufficiently specific to invite correct recall.

Another approach would be to ask participants to maintain a diary of daily sexual-activity. However, there are problems with this as well. Because it takes a special type of participant to be willing to comply, the potential participant pool may become too restrictive, and thus introduce selection bias that would be difficult to measure. It is unlikely that women at high risk for infection, often living difficult and disrupted lives, would be willing or even able to maintain a diary. Timeliness and accuracy of data entry would be uncertain. Moreover, the very act of recording sexual activity and condom-use behaviour may in itself constitute an intervention, similar to food diaries for the overweight. Thus, results probably would not be generalizable to a broader population.

If the objective of a given intervention is to change a specific behaviour that may contribute to reduced infection rates, such as consistent condom use, it would be sufficient to focus on this behaviour, and to examine self-reported behaviour regarding this outcome. However, if the objective is to reduce infection rates, a more holistic approach is required. Given the complex relationship between behaviour and disease incidence, such interventions must focus on changing several behaviours. For example, it is not sufficient to increase condom use or rates of mutual monogamy, if having sex with an untreated partner is neglected. It is not surprising that, when included as a variable, having sex/unprotected sex with an untreated or incompletely treated partner is the strongest predictor of infection.[1,12,14,15] Mutual monogamy is not protective if the partner remains infectious. On the other hand, mutual monogamy, coupled with having a fully treated partner, is exceedingly protective. When the results of Project SAFE were first published,[1] intervention efficacy was attributed to the multiplicity of behaviours addressed, from health-seeking behaviour and adherence to treatment protocols to a focus on correct, consistent condom use, and male–female relationships. Because different aspects of behaviour and circumstances interact, it is important to influence several key factors simultaneously. It is also important to impress upon intervention participants the importance of exercising judgment in their decision-making processes. For example, if the realities of their lives make them likely to choose multiple or risky partners, it is especially important for them to be vigilant about consistent and correct condom use. Intervention participants can also learn the importance of not having unprotected sex with a partner until she knows he is not infected.

In order to develop measures of sexual behaviour that are meaningful with respect to likelihood of infection, it is critical to include biological parameters. It is important to examine behavioural measures similar to those used in Project SAFE in the context of other studies to determine if their utility is broadly based. For example, in the Project SAFE study population, the question concerning checking that the penis was fully covered was strongly related to new infection. This was not surprising, since prior exploratory work suggested that it would be useful. This may not be the case in other populations. This also speaks to the importance of knowing one's target population.

Conclusion

It has been shown that simple behaviours, commonly addressed and measured in isolation, are often unrelated to infection rates. The link between behaviour and biology is clarified when behavioural measures incorporate context, and are considered simultaneously. Both the development of interventions, and evaluation of their efficacy, must reflect this complex interplay among sexual risk behaviours and infection.

References

1. Shain, R.N., Piper, J.M., Newton, E.R., Perdue, S.T., Ramos, R., Champion, J.D., and Guerra, F.A. (1999) A randomised, controlled trial of a behavioural intervention to prevent sexually transmitted disease among minority women. *New Engl J Med*, **340**, 93–100.

2. Kamb, M.L., Fishbein, M., Douglas, J.M., Rhodes, F., Rogers, J., Bolan, G., Zenilman, J., *et al.* (1998) Efficacy of risk-reduction counselling to prevent human immunodeficiency virus and sexually transmitted diseases. *JAMA*, **280**, 1161–7.

3. The National Institute of Mental Health (NIMH) Multisite HIV Prevention Trial Group. (1998) The NIMH Multisite HIV Prevention Trial: reducing HIV sexual risk behaviour. *Science*, **280**, 1889–94.

4. Boyer, C.B., Barrett, D.C., Peterman, T.A., and Bolan, G. (1997) Sexually transmitted disease (STD) and HIV risk in heterosexual adults attending a public STD clinic: evaluation of a randomised controlled behavioural risk-reduction intervention trial. *AIDS*, **11**, 359–67.

5. Jemmott, J.B., Jemmott, L.S., and Fong, G.T. (1998) Abstinence and safer sex HIV risk reduction interventions for African American adolescents: a randomized controlled trial. *JAMA*, **279**, 1529–36.

6. Kelly, J.A., Murphy, D.A., Washington, C.D., *et al.* (1994) The effects of HIV/AIDS intervention groups for high-risk women in urban clinics. *Am J Public Health*, **84**, 1918–22.

7. DiClemente, R.J. and Wingood, G.M. (1995) A randomized controlled trial of an HIV sexual risk-reduction intervention for young African-American women. *JAMA*, **274**, 1271–6.

8. Imrie, J., Stephenson, J.M., Cowan, F.M., Wanigaratne, S., Billington, A.J., Copas, A.J., French, L., French, P.D., and Johnson, A.M. (2001) A cognitive behavioural intervention to reduce sexually transmitted infections among gay men: randomised trial. *Br Med J*, **322**, 1451–56.

9. Branson, B.M., Barrett, D.C., Peterman, T.A., and Bolan, G. (1998) Group counselling to prevent sexually transmitted disease and HIV: a randomised controlled trial. *Sex Transm Dis*, **25**, 553–60.

10. Orr, D.P., Langefeld, C.D., Katz, B.P., and Caine, V.A. (1996) Behavioural intervention to increase condom use among high-risk female adolescents. *J Pediatr*, **128**, 288–95.

11. Stephenson, J., Imrie, J., and Sutton, S.R. (2000) Rigorous trials of sexual behaviour interventions in STD/HIV prevention: what can we learn from them? *AIDS*, **14**(suppl. 3): S115–S124.

12. Shain, R.N., Perdue, S., Piper, J.M., Holden, A., Dimmitt-Champion, J., Newton, E.R., *et al.* (1999) Sexual risk-reduction behaviours amenable to intervention: the importance of context. 13th Meeting of the International Society for Sexually Transmitted Diseases Research. Denver CO, USA, 11–14 July 1999, Abstract No. 001.

13. Shain, R.N., Piper, J.M., Newton, E.R., Perdue, S., Champion, J., Holden, A., *et al.* (1997) A controlled randomised trial of a risk-reduction intervention: behaviours contributing to reduced infection rates at 12 months' follow-up. *12th Meeting of the International Society for Sexually Transmitted Diseases Research*. Seville, Spain, 19–22 October 1997, Abstract O202.

14. Shain, R.N., Perdue, S.T., Piper, J., Holden, A.E.C., Champion, J.D., and Newton, E.R. (2002) Behaviours changed by intervention are associated with reduced STD recurrence—the importance of context in measurement, *Sex Transm Dis*, **29**(9), 520–9.

15. Perdue, S.T., Sahin, R.N., Piper, J.M., Holden, A., Dimmitt-Champion, J., Newton, E.R., *et al.* (1999) Risk-reduction index for behaviours amenable to intervention. *13th Meeting of the International Society for Sexually Transmitted Diseases Research*. Denver CO, USA, 11–14 July 1999, Abstract No. 001.

16. Peterman, T.A., Lin, L.S., Newman, D.R., Kamb, M.L., Bolan, G., Zenilman, J., Douglas Jr, J.M., Rogers, J., and Malotte, C.K., for the Project RESPECT Study Group. (2000) Does measured behaviour reflect STD risk? An analysis of data from a randomized controlled behavioural intervention study. *Sex Transm Dis*, **27**(8), 446–51.

17. Peterman, T.A., Lin, L., Newman, D., Kamb, M.L., Bolan, G., Zenilman, J., *et al.* (1997) Association between behaviour change and STD incidence? *12th Meeting of the International Society for Sexually Transmitted Diseases Research*. Seville, Spain, 19–22 October 1997, Abstract P603.

18. De Vincenzi, I., for the European Study Group on Heterosexual Transmission of HIV. (1994) A longitudinal study of human immunodeficiency virus transmission by heterosexual partners. *New Engl J Med*, **331**(6), 341–6.

19. Aral, S.O. and Peterman, T. (1996) Measuring the outcomes of behavioural interventions for STD/HIV prevention. *Int J STD AIDS*, **7**(suppl. 2), 30–8.

20. O'Leary, A., DiClemente, R.J., and Aral, S.O. (1997) Reflections on the design and reporting of STD/HIV behavioural interventions research. *AIDS Educ Prev*, **9**, 1–5.

21. Zenilman, J.M., Weisman, C.S., Rompalo, A.M., Ellish, N., Upchurch, D.M., Hook, E.W., and Celentano, D. (1995) Condom use to prevent incident STDs: the validity of self-reported condom use. *Sex Transm Dis*, **22**(1), 15–21.

22. Turner, C.F. and Miller, H.G. (1997) Zenilman's anomaly reconsidered: fallible reports, Ceteris Paribus, and other hypotheses. *Sex Transm Dis*, **24**(9), 522–7.

23. Fishbein, M. and Pequegnat, W. (2000) Evaluating AIDS prevention interventions using behavioural and biological outcome measures. *Sex Transm Dis*, **27**(2), 101–10.

24. Fishbein, M. and Jarvis, B. (2000) Failure to find a behavioural surrogate for STD incidence—what does it really mean? *Sex Transm Dis*, **27**(8), 452–5.

25. Pequegnat, W., Fishbein, M., Celentano, D., Ehrhardt, A., Garnett, G., Holtgrave, D., Jaccard, J., Schachter, J., and Zenilman, J. (2000) NIMH/APPC workgroup on a behavioural and biological outcomes in HIV/STD prevention studies: a position statement. *Sex Transm Dis*, **27**(3), 127–32.

26. Richens, J., Imrie, J., and Copas, A. (2000) Condoms and seat belts: the parallels and the lessons. *Lancet*, **355**(9201), 400–3.

27. Shain, R.N., Piper, J.M., Perdue, S., Holden, A., Champion, J.D., and Guerra, F. (2001) Behavioural intervention reduces rates of chlamydia and/or gonorrhea among minority women at 12 and 24 months' follow-up. *International Congress of Sexually Transmitted Infections*, ISSTDR/IUSTI. Berlin, Germany, 24–27 June 2001, p. 80.

Chapter 10

Unpacking the 'black box': the importance of process data to explain outcomes

Daniel Wight and Angela Obasi

Introduction

Discussion about methodologies and effectiveness evaluation frequently becomes polarized between positivist approaches (i.e. quantitative, outcome-orientated research), and other approaches variously labelled interpretivist, phenomenological or relativist (i.e. qualitative, process-orientated research). However, this dichotomy was challenged at least thirty years ago,[1] and the debates it generates now are increasingly unhelpful and tedious.[2] In this chapter, we hope to illustrate how the research design of evaluations can be strengthened by combining elements of different epistemological approaches. This pluralist position has been said to stem from the 'realist' tradition in the philosophy of science.[2]

We are committed to the rigorous evaluation of intervention outcomes, and consider that, if the nature of the intervention, target group and social context allow, this is best done through a randomized controlled trial (RCT). However, there are serious problems with evaluations that focus exclusively on outcomes. Amongst the many critiques[2–6] six appear to be particularly important.

1. Elaborate and expensive outcome studies are sometimes established to evaluate an intervention that has been poorly designed and developed. If, as is likely, the outcomes then suggest it is not effective, it will mean a huge waste of resources, and can lead to the false assumption that any intervention in this area would fail.

2. Conventional RCTs compare groups according to their initial allocation, irrespective of what intervention they did, in fact, receive: in drug trial parlance an 'intention-to-treat' analysis. Any other analysis loses the strict balance between arms, which is the main rationale of an RCT. However this emphasis on intention-to-analysis can lead to false conclusions.

For instance a negative outcome might be assumed to be due to an inadequate intervention rather than, for example, poor delivery or a lack of contrast between the interventions received in each arm of the trial.

3. Outcome evaluations do little to improve our understanding of the mechanisms by which an intervention is supposed to work, and thus fail to inform the further development of effective interventions.[2]

4. An RCT of a complex programme with several components will not, in itself, allow one to distinguish which components were a success or failure.

5. Outcome evaluations do not investigate the crucial contextual factors that might facilitate or prevent the success of an intervention: unless this is known it is difficult to ensure their replication in other settings.[2]

6. Investigating the impact of an intervention in aggregate, which is often essential to have sufficient statistical power, does not explore differential effects within the target group. Yet, many programmes have heterogeneous effects and aggregation may obscure more than it reveals.[7]

Trials employing intention-to-treat analyses are 'pragmatic' (i.e. they seek to answer the question 'Which programme should we adopt?'), rather than 'explanatory' (i.e. aimed at understanding).[8] The former do not attempt to explain the essential features of an intervention's success, such as the mechanism by which it worked and context in which this was possible. Indeed, 'It is characteristic of the pragmatic approach that the treatments are flexibly defined and "absorb" into themselves the contexts in which they are administered (see Ref. 8, p. 638).' This may lead to the replication of an apparently effective intervention in a different setting where it is likely to fail. A good illustration (see Chapter 13) is the attempt to adapt for Glasgow, Scotland, the 'Gay Heroes' peer-education programme that had been demonstrated to have reduced unsafe sex amongst gay men in the United States.[9] The failure of the intervention in Glasgow was attributed largely to the different social context, particularly a reluctance to discuss sexual practices in gay bars and clubs, and less urgent concern about the HIV epidemic than a decade earlier—before the wide spread introduction of highly active antiretroviral therapy (HAART).[10] Neither of these crucial contextual factors had been documented in the evaluation by Kelly et al.[9]

Many of those who advance these criticisms of RCTs conclude, more or less explicitly, that randomized controlled trials of social interventions are rarely, if ever, appropriate.[6] However, we consider it should be possible to combine the strengths of a randomized approach (see Chapters 1 and 3) with the 'theory-driven' or 'realistic' approach that has been advocated by Pawson and Tilley.[2]

The essence of this approach is to base the outcome evaluation on a thorough understanding of the process of the intervention and to complement it with the collection of good process data, in particular using Pawson and Tilley's formula: 'Outcomes = Mechanism + Context'.[2] In short, an unintelligible intervention, or 'black box', has to be unpacked.

This is illustrated through two RCTs currently under analysis in Scotland and Tanzania. Following an outline of the projects, the chapter discusses four key intervention factors that can be of critical importance in interpreting outcome evaluations. These factors are: (1) the extent and quality of intervention delivery; (2) the mechanism; (3) the context; and, (4) the response of the target group. Finally, we consider some key problems with process evaluations and how process and outcome data can be integrated.

Two case studies: SHARE and MEMA kwa Vijana

The SHARE study: eastern Scotland

In 1993, an inter-disciplinary group of researchers set about developing a teacher-delivered sex education programme for 13–15-year-olds with the intention of rigorously evaluating it. Following a preliminary feasibility study, a programme was developed called 'SHARE: Sexual Health and Relationships—Safe, Happy and Responsible', intended to improve the quality of young people's sexual relationships, reduce unsafe sex and reduce unwanted pregnancies. The programme was based on an understanding of the possible mechanism for behavioural change that came from a combination of theories from social psychology (primarily the Theory of Planned Behaviour), and sociology (interactionism and feminism).[11] SHARE was developed over two years, involving two detailed pilots, each in four schools, and extensive consultation with practitioners, researchers and the education establishment.[12] It comprises a five day teacher training course and a 20 session pack to be delivered in the third and fourth years of secondary school. The course takes a harm reduction approach and differs from conventional school sex education by attempting to develop sexual negotiation and condom use skills, primarily through the use of interactive video.

The SHARE trial started in 1996. Twenty-five schools in eastern Scotland were randomly allocated either to deliver SHARE or to continue with their existing sex education. The latter varied between seven and twelve lessons over the two years and consisted primarily of information provision and discussion. A total of 7630 pupils were followed from ages 13–14 (at baseline) to ages 15–16 (roughly six months post-programme) using self-completion questionnaires.

When compared with those receiving conventional sex education, at six months post-intervention SHARE recipients demonstrated:

♦ higher satisfaction with their sex education,

♦ greater practical sexual health knowledge,

♦ an improvement in the quality of sexual relationships in respect to one measure only,

♦ lack of regret, and

♦ no change in any of the reported behavioural measures.[13]

Process data were collected through in-depth interviews with pupils and teachers, pupil group discussions, observation of lessons and training, self-completion teacher lesson forms and teacher and pupil questionnaires.

It is planned to follow the cohorts for a further four years to the age of 20. At that point, it should be possible to evaluate the impact of the programme on cumulative abortion rates, using National Health Service data—an outcome measure that is not subject to reporting bias or attrition.

The MEMA kwa Vijana (Good Things for Young People) study: northern Tanzania

The gravity of the HIV epidemic in sub-Saharan Africa has been well described, as has the urgency to develop and evaluate reproductive health interventions for young people.[14,15] However, this urgency precludes the luxury of many years of careful development. In reality, programmes are often subjected to an outcome evaluation while still being modified through an iterative process of formative evaluation. The MEMA randomized trial is evaluating just such a 'real world' scenario.

MEMA kwa Vijana is a three-year adolescent reproductive health programme for 15–19 year olds in rural northern Tanzania.[16] Using a combination of rational motivational and social learning theories,[17,18] the intervention aims to reduce the incidence of HIV, other sexually transmitted infections (STIs) and unwanted pregnancy by improving reproductive health knowledge, teaching skills to promote behavioural change, increasing health service uptake and addressing some of the contextual factors affecting adolescent reproductive health.[19] The intervention in the MEMA kwa Vijana study has four main components: (1) raising community awareness and support; (2) teacher-led, peer-assisted skills-based education in the last three years of primary school; (3) condom social marketing by peers; and, (4) provision of youth friendly health services. The programme is implemented through existing government structures and is designed to be sustainable and reproducible on a large scale in resource poor settings.

Development of the first year of the teacher-led programme began in 1997. This involved reviews of local and international best practice materials and strategies,[11,20–22] reviewing evaluations of local programmes,[23,24] and pre-testing of the programme in three schools. The modified programme was then pilot-tested in a further six schools in order to assess feasibility, acceptability and appropriateness of the programme as well as its impact on pupil knowledge, using observation, questionnaires and group discussions.[25] Teachers received five days' training each year and the curriculum is distinguished by the inclusion of elected peer-educators, who perform mini-dramas as discussion starters in the classroom, and the active use of role-play to model key skills.

Before implementation, community stake-holders including parents, teachers, government officials, community and religious leaders, elected advisory committees to monitor intervention activities at local level, and elect community peer-educators. Health workers received six days' participatory training focusing on empathy, confidentiality, and the rights of young people to access health services.

During the three-year trial, data have been collected via observations of teaching and clinic sessions, and practitioner questionnaires, report forms and group discussions. These have informed the development of teacher guides for each school year and a refresher training course for health workers. Finally, towards the end of the first year of the trial, a peer condom social marketing initiative was developed, piloted and implemented in response to demand in the intervention communities.

Twenty 'communities' have been randomized to receive either the intervention or continue with the existing minimal sex education and sexual health service provision. Each intervention community is roughly equivalent to a ward, which is the smallest unit of local government made up of an average of six villages. These vary between lakeside fishing villages, busy roadside settlements, mining communities and traditional inland farming areas. The intervention began in 63 villages in January 1999. Its impact on HIV, genital herpes, gonorrhoea, chlamydia, pregnancy, and reported behaviour is being evaluated over three years in a cohort of 9299 pupils aged 14 and over at recruitment.[26] The final evaluation survey began in October 2001.

The ongoing development of the intervention throughout the trial, plus the need to monitor each component, has necessitated repeated field visits by the implementation team. This has provided detailed, rich and systematic data that allow us to assess which components and modifications were of most value in generating the final outcomes. Examples from these two studies are used to illustrate the key points in the remainder of the chapter.

Extent and quality of programme delivery

To interpret outcome findings it is essential to know something about the extent and quality of delivery of the intervention. In a well-organized programme this information would be collected largely through routine monitoring by the practitioners themselves. Where a new intervention is being compared with standard procedures in the control group, it is also important to know what this standard consists of and how well it was delivered.

Illustrations from the SHARE study

Information that had already been collected about the extent and quality of delivery of the programme has been particularly important in the SHARE study because the outcomes from an intention-to-treat analysis showed no behavioural effect of the intervention. An obvious interpretation is that the programme failed, but the results might also be attributed to poor delivery or a failure of the research design to demonstrate an effect.[13] By taking into account the extent and quality of the SHARE intervention delivery, and the nature of sex education programmes in the control schools, it was possible to conduct an 'on-treatment' analysis that compares groups according to the intervention that they actually received, rather than that to which they were allocated.

Before looking at the outcomes by arm of the trial or by school, classes were dichotomized into whether they were 'on treatment' or not, drawing on teachers' lesson forms, in-depth interviews, curricular materials and lesson observations. To be 'on treatment' required that:

+ pupils received at least 15/20 sessions;
+ there were appropriate exercises to develop skills in negotiation and condom use, and inform pupils about accessing local services; and
+ there was no evidence that the quality of teaching was insufficient to learn anything.

Sex education programmes in the control schools were also classified on this basis, since some might have also met these criteria.

The on-treatment approach inevitably loses the balance between arms of the trial because the delivery factors are most unlikely to be distributed evenly. Therefore multi-variate analysis was necessary to control for the independent variables by which the arms of the trial had originally been balanced (e.g. the socio-demographic characteristics of school catchments), and results had to be presented in odds ratios. The on-treatment analysis ascertained that the trial outcomes were not attributable to the poor delivery of the intervention nor to the lack of contrast with the sex education in the control schools. Although the intention-to-treat analysis provided an outcome finding more applicable to the real world, and thus to policy makers, little was explained by such a pragmatic trial without an 'on-treatment' analysis.

Illustrations from the MEMA study

The extent and quality of delivery of each of the four components of the MEMA intervention were assessed through routine collection of detailed quantitative information by the research team, as part of the ongoing formative evaluation. These data included information on the number of practitioners trained, practitioner transfers and losses, teaching sessions covered, patients seen, and so on. The quality of intervention delivery was also investigated by researchers presenting themselves as patients at health services,[27] through external, in-depth, qualitative evaluations of teacher training and classroom sessions, peer training,[28] and peer education.[29]

Finally, other government and non-government organization sexual health initiatives began in the trial communities during the study period. Two surveys are monitoring these activities so that a judgement can be made as to the degree of contrast between intervention and control groups in their exposure to these initiatives.

Mechanism of interventions

In conventional clinical trials, the mechanism by which the intervention is assumed to work has been established by basic biological research and Phase I and II trials before the RCT starts (see Chapter 5). However, with behavioural interventions the mechanisms by which they are meant to operate are generally far less clearly understood. Not only is preparatory research rarely as systematic and rigorous as Phase I and II trials, but the mechanisms are usually social or socio-psychological, rather than biological. Compared with the body there is far less consensus on the workings of the social world, where understanding, such as it exists, tends to be rougher, more uncertain and contingent.[7]

Ideally, the design of an intervention is based on some understanding of the mechanism by which it is meant to work, and this is further clarified and confirmed during the intervention's development. In practice, however, programme development is often extremely rushed or researchers adopt a pre-existing programme and the mechanism is implicit and/or only vaguely understood. Collecting data to understand how the programme is working, or why it is not, is then essential if the trial is to contribute to the development of more effective interventions. Even when the postulated mechanism has been well identified before the trial, it is still useful to investigate whether it is working as predicted.

Illustrations from the SHARE study

The eclectic theoretical basis for SHARE identified various ways in which the programme should have impacted on behaviour.[11] One of the objectives of the evaluation was to explore whether these mechanisms worked as intended, both through qualitative and quantitative research (in particular cognition scales, which might be considered intermediate outcomes). Teacher and pupil interviews and the observation of lessons and teacher training suggested why the intended mechanisms might have failed. Here, we consider just one, that of skills development, which according to the Theory of Planned Behaviour could be achieved by enhancing self-efficacy through modelling other's behaviour, planning and rehearsing.[17] With SHARE, however, the time available might have been inadequate to model behaviour, and some teachers were rather unclear about the theoretical approach or found skills-based exercises particularly difficult to deliver. Many pupils were not motivated to acquire new skills. In most successful behavioural programmes, participation is voluntary whereas school sex education is compulsory and pupils cannot choose when to attend in relation to their personal lives. Furthermore, it comes within social education, a non-examined subject, in which pupils expect to be able to relax and many are unwilling to actively participate if it involves an effort.

Illustrations from the MEMA study

The MEMA intervention was informed by assumptions of rational decision-making and patterns of social influence based on models developed from experience in the developed world. How applicable these models are to the developing world is simply not known.[19,30] It is critical to investigate how the proposed mechanisms (e.g. modelling of behaviour through role-play, or changing perceived norms through the use of drama), really work in cultures where teachers are unfamiliar with interactive teaching strategies and where public discussion of sexual matters may in itself be stigmatizing, regardless of positive messages. Information about these factors has been collected through classroom observations, teacher report forms and interviews with pupils, peer-educators, teachers, head teachers, health workers, and parents.

Context of intervention

Closely related to the mechanism of the intervention is the context necessary for it to work. Process evaluations need to investigate the enabling and impeding influences on delivery and impact, in order to understand better the necessary conditions for interventions to be effective. Having a grasp of these contextual factors, as well as the mechanism by which the programme works, is essential to know how transferable a successful intervention is likely to be to other populations or countries.[2]

Illustrations from the SHARE study

Many data were collected concerning the context of the SHARE programme, and again this has provided possible explanations for the outcome findings. At classroom level, pupil interviews and group discussions threw light on those aspects of classroom relationships necessary for pupils to feel confident to engage in the lesson: the teachers' control of their classes, their friendliness towards pupils, their treatment of the topic as fun and the trust between pupils.[31] At the school level, pre-requisites for SHARE to be delivered well were: senior management support, a coherent team, an enthusiastic co-ordinator and sufficiently long lessons.[32] Quantitative data from the trial also help to explain and understand the context. Multi-level analysis of the outcomes highlights the importance of parental influence, and shows that there is a clear 'school effect' on sexual behaviour. It is hoped that the contextual data on schools will allow this latter finding to be explained.

Illustrations from the MEMA study

The contextual factors in northern Tanzania are, if anything, more complex and less well understood than in the case of eastern Scotland. Many background circumstances taken for granted in the developed world—availability of classrooms, class sizes under fifty, high levels of attendance and literacy, or even regular payment of teachers' salary—are extremely variable and sometimes non-existent in resource poor settings. Poverty can also have a profound impact on important aspects of the intervention process. For example, the apparently minor incentives that peer-educators receive, such as meals during training or T-shirts, may be so significant as to undermine their status as 'peers' and hence their validity as role models or educators.[29] The impact of these factors on the implementation of the intervention is crucial to understanding its feasibility and transferability.

The health and education systems through which the MEMA programme was implemented have their own very different cultures. Inherent conservatism within the education system constrained the design of the intervention and may have had a negative impact on coverage and delivery.[33] However, the inclusion of entire schools was fundamental to the evaluation design and so effective means to minimize resistance had to be found. Understanding the culture of the institutions that deliver an intervention is crucial to its design and to maximizing its implementation.

Finally, the attitudes of the host communities, particularly to the open discussion of sexual matters, will necessarily affect intervention success. These attitudes vary considerably and addressing particular individuals or groups within the community can have a significant impact on the success of the implementation. For example, in one community, a religious group severely disrupted implementation of the programme by condemning the discussion of sexual matters in class and ceremonially burning a project T-shirt. However, following discussions with the researchers, a senior member of the group agreed to participate in some of the MEMA activities and the hostility was reversed.

Understanding such contextual factors is probably more difficult in the developing world because of the limited resources for social research and the scarcity of indigenous researchers. It was particularly challenging within the MEMA programme since this involved several sectors and was delivered in ten different communities. However, this very complexity provides an opportunity to explore the means by which these contextual circumstances impact on the implementation of the different components of the programme.

Differential response of target group

If a behavioural intervention is to work, it has to reach its target audience and they have to be receptive. However, in trials with sufficient statistical power to demonstrate a modest effect of an intervention, the target audience is likely to be heterogeneous, particularly in cluster randomized trials. Some sub-groups are almost certainly going to be more receptive to the intervention than others, and identifying what works for whom is important in understanding the effectiveness of the overall programme.[2]

Illustrations from the SHARE study

In the SHARE study pupils' differential response to the programme was explored through both process data, particularly those from lesson observations and pupil interviews, and through outcome data. Gender differences in response to sex education are already well established and reviews have highlighted the importance of prior sexual experience in shaping the effectiveness of programmes.[34-36] The sample size was adequate to analyse the outcomes according to such sub-groups (i.e. young women vs young men, previously sexually experienced vs non-experienced). However, hypotheses about sub-groups should, ideally, be formulated in advance to ensure sufficient power to conduct the sub-group analysis without the risk of generating false positives from post-hoc data dredging.

Illustrations from MEMA study

Young people's experience of, and response to, the MEMA programme differ greatly according to their gender and status as a pupil, peer-educator or youth in the community. These issues have been explored through interviews, observation and questionnaires. The influence of classroom culture on the gendered experience of the intervention is particularly striking. A range of factors, from the paucity of female teachers to girls' traditional inhibition in participating in mixed group discussions or drama, all have an impact on how girls experience the intervention relative to their male counterparts.[29]

Problems with process evaluation

While process evaluation is an essential complement to outcome evaluation, it is important to acknowledge the problems that process evaluations may themselves generate. These are exacerbated when, as is often the case with behavioural interventions in the developing world, most process data are collected by the implementation team. The problems may be particularly acute in intensive formative evaluations such as that in the MEMA study.

Evaluation and reporting bias

In most sexual health intervention trials, including both SHARE and MEMA, key members of the evaluation team have previously been involved in the design of the intervention and therefore have an interest in demonstrating its effectiveness. Ideally, the evaluation team would be entirely distinct from those who developed the intervention. A greater problem exists when the implementation team also collect the process data. Their deep involvement may lead them to judge the success or failure of activities either too harshly or too leniently. Similarly teachers, health workers and peer-educators develop relationships with their trainers and supervisors over time that will necessarily impact on the way they report their activities to them.

Evaluation as intervention

In certain circumstances, the process evaluation of a programme can itself become an intervention. For instance, evaluative group discussions with teachers may motivate them to perform to levels that would not have been achieved otherwise. This is particularly important in developing countries where there may be virtually no provision in the control groups, and so no possibility of balancing the evaluation impact across arms. The question then arises as to how much of the intervention impact is due to the process of its evaluation, a question probably best answered through a 'Solomon four-group design',[37] in which there is a two-by-two design to the trial with four groups allocated to either intervention or non-intervention arms, and to either minimum or maximum evaluation arms.

Misinterpretation

Process data are often qualitative and so their collection and analysis is less standardised than outcome or quantitative data. Consequently, they are more prone to observer- and reporter-biases and there is a danger that factors identified during the process evaluation which seem to be intuitively important may turn out not to be so. This highlights the value of integrating process and outcome data.

Integration of process and outcome data

Although process findings can be valuable in their own right, unless they are analysed in conjunction with outcome findings of a trial they are of no greater value than those generated from smaller scale, exclusively process evaluations. This raises the question of how process and outcome data should be combined and whether outcome findings can be used to understand processes better, as well as vice versa.

Unless the process or the outcome data is privileged in epistemological terms, each is likely to influence the analysis of the other. The sequence in which this is done does not seem important except that, since much of the process data is qualitative, there is probably a greater danger of bias in interpreting it. For instance, if the outcome data suggest that the programme was ineffective in one particular school, when analysing interview and observational data on teacher's motivation, it is possible that signs of low motivation are over-interpreted in this school. Therefore, the most rigorous way of using the process data to interpret outcomes is to identify the key process factors likely to affect the outcomes before analysing the outcome data. With each factor one would then compute a score for each unit of analysis, such as school or community. This would create independent quantitative variables that could be used in analysing the outcome data. The categorization of classes as 'on' or 'off' treatment in the SHARE trial, discussed above, is an example of this. Similarly, initial process data from the MEMA study indicate that there are differences in local government management at district level that may have had a profound impact on intervention implementation. These will be characterized in advance and their impact on outcomes assessed.

It is worth noting that some process data may stem from the incorrect assumptions of participants in the intervention about its outcomes. For instance, participants in 'Scared Straight' programmes, in which young offenders visit long-term prison inmates in order to be discouraged from a life of crime, generally assume the programmes to be effective and speak about them very positively, yet, randomized trials demonstrate that they are not effective.[38]

Outcome findings can also inform the interpretation of processes. We have already mentioned that 'school effects' were identified from the SHARE outcome data, and these will shape the analysis of process data. Similar important effects may be seen in the MEMA study outcomes.

Conclusion

The collection of good process data should overcome many of the limitations of experimental evaluations that rely exclusively on outcomes. Good process data can establish whether the intervention is delivered as intended and to what extent it contrasts with programmes in the control arm. They can improve our understanding of the mechanisms through which the intervention is meant to work, and identify which elements of a complex intervention are best delivered and have the best response from the target group. Furthermore, process data can throw light on the crucial contextual factors that facilitate or prevent the success of the intervention and can explore how different sections of the target group respond to the intervention.

However, recognizing the importance of these process factors also means acknowledging their importance in the design and development of the intervention before beginning the trial. A process evaluation should not be seen as a substitute for careful formative evaluation that clarifies the mechanisms of the intervention and the context it requires. Another limitation of process evaluations is that they can only throw light on, but not resolve, which elements of a complex intervention seem to be most effective. To establish this clearly would require separate outcome evaluations, such as trials with multiple arms.

Although there is a general assumption that outcome evaluations exclusively involve quantitative methods and process evaluations qualitative methods, by drawing on contrasting epistemological approaches it is possible to benefit from combining quantitative and qualitative methods within both forms of evaluation. Both the SHARE and MEMA studies have included in-depth interviews as part of their outcome evaluations, to help validate the self-reported behavioural data,[39] and to explore more complex issues. The effectiveness of the MEMA intervention is also being evaluated through participant observation. Equally, the process evaluations in both studies have combined quantitative and qualitative methods.

We have argued that by combining elements of different epistemological approaches, the research design of experimental evaluations can be strengthened. Trials of interventions in the social world should attempt to explain the essential features of the intervention's success or failure, such as the quality of delivery, the mechanism by which the programme is supposed to work and the context necessary for this to be possible. Without 'unpacking the black box' in such a way, the outcomes of an experimental evaluation are of little value since they cannot be explained.

Acknowledgements

We would like to thank our colleagues for their contributions to these arguments over a long period of time, and in particular to thank the following for their detailed comments on previous drafts: Chris Bonell, Katie Buston, Sally Macintyre, Mark Petticrew, David Ross and Erica Wimbush. The SHARE trial has been supported by the UK Medical Research Council, and the development of the programme was funded by the Health Education Board for Scotland. The MEMA kwa Vijana trial is a collaboration between the Tanzanian National Institute for Medical Research (NIMR), the African Medical and Research Foundation (AMREF), the London School of Hygiene and Tropical Medicine (LSHTM), and the Ministries of Health and of Education and Culture of the Government of Tanzania, and has been funded by the European Union, the UK Medical Research Council, and UK Department for International Development.

References

1. Berger, P. and Luckmann, T. (1966) *The Social Construction of Reality*. Anchor Books, New York.

2. Pawson, R. and Tilley, N. (1997) *Realistic Evaluation*. Sage, London.

3. Tones, K. (1997) Beyond the randomised controlled trial: a case for 'judicial' review. *Health Educ Res*, **12**, i–iv.

4. Kippax, S. and Van den Ven, P. (1998) An epidemic of orthodoxy? Design and methodology in the evaluation of the effectiveness of HIV health promotion. *Crit Public Health*, **8**, 371–86.

5. Van den Ven, P. and Aggleton, P. (1999) What constitutes evidence in HIV/AIDS education? *Health Educ Res*, **14**, 461–71.

6. Springett, J. (2001) Practical guidance on evaluating health promotion. WHO-Euro Working Group on the Evaluation of Health Promotion.

7. Davies, H., Nutley, S., and Tilley, N. (2000) Debates on the role of experimentation. In: Davies, H., Nutley, S., and Smith, P. (eds) *What Works?*, Policy Press.

8. Schwarz, D. and Lellouch, J. (1967) Explanatory and pragmatic attitudes in clinical trials. *J Chronic Dis*, **20**, 637–48.

9. Kelly, J.A., Murphy, D.A., Sikkema, K.J., McAuliffe, T.L., Roffman, R.A., Solomon, L.J., *et al.* (1997) Randomised, controlled, community-level HIV-prevention intervention for sexual-risk behaviour among homosexual men in US cities. *Lancet*, **350**, 1500–5.

10. Flowers, P., Hart, G.J., Williamson, L.M., Frankis, J.S., and Der, G.J. (2002) Does bar-based peer-led sexual health promotion have a community-level effect amongst gay men in Scotland? *Int J STD AIDS*, **13**, 102–8.

11. Wight, D., Abraham, C., and Scott, S. (1998) Towards a psycho-social framework for sexual health promotion. *Health Educ Res*, **13**, 317–30.

12. Wight, D. and Abraham, C. (2000) From psycho-social theory to sustainable classroom practice: developing a research-based teacher-delivered sex education programme. *Health Educ Res*, **15**, 25–38.

13. Wight, D., Raab, G., Henderson, M., Abraham, C., Buston, K., Hart, G., and Scott, S. (2002) The limits of teacher-delivered sex education: interim behavioural outcomes from a randomised trial. *Br Med J*, **324**, 1430–3.

14. UNAIDS. (2000) Report on the Global HIV/AIDS Epidemic. Geneva, Switzerland.

15. World Health Organization. (1993) Sexually Transmitted Diseases Among Adolescents in Developing Countries. WHO, Geneva.

16. Nyamwaya, D., Bisecko, S., Garbone, R., Gavyole, A., Grosskurth, H., Hayes, R., *et al.* (1997) Prevention of HIV infection and enhancement of reproductive health among adolescents in rural Tanzania: A community randomised trial. Part 1: Rationale & Design of the intervention. *12th Meeting of the International Society of Sexually Transmitted Diseases Research*. Seville, Spain, 19–22 October 1997, Abstract No. S43.

17. Ajzen, I. and Fishbein, M. (1980) Understanding attitudes and predicting social behaviour. Prentice-Hall, Englewood Cliffs, NJ, USA.

18. Bandura, A. (1977) Self-efficacy: towards a unifying theory of behavioural change. *Psychol Rev*, **84**, 191–215.

19. Hughes, J. and McCauley, A.P. (1998) Improving the fit: Adolescents' needs and future programs for sexual and reproductive health in developing countries. *Stud Fam Plann*, **29**, 233–45.

20. World Health Organization. (1994) School Health Education to Prevent AIDS and STD: A Resource Package for Curriculum Planners. WHO/GPA/PRV/94.6 a–c, WHO, Geneva.

21. Kirby, D., Short, L., Collins, J., Rugg, D., Kolbe, L., Howard, M., *et al.* (1994) School-based programmes to reduce sexual risk behaviours: a review of effectiveness. *Public Health Rep*, **109**, 339–60.

22. Mgalla, Z. and Obasi, A. (1997) *National Workshop on AIDS Preventative Education in Schools.* 5–7 May 1997, Dar es Salaam, Tanzania.

23. Plummer, M. (1994) Consultancy Report: Development, Implementation and Evaluation of a Secondary School Peer AIDS Education Programme. Kuleana Centre for Children's Rights and AIDS Action, Mwanza, Tanzania.

24. Plummer, M.L. and Maswe, M. (1998) Evaluation Report for the TANESA Primary School Peer Health Education Programme. Project to Support AIDS Control in Mwanza Region. Mwanza, Tanzania, Tanzania-Netherlands.

25. Chima, K., Obasi, A., Cleophas-Frisch, B., Ross, D.A., and Mujaya, B. (1999) Impact of a teacher-led health intervention on pupil knowledge in primary schools in Mwanza, Tanzania. *13th Meeting of the International Society for Sexually Transmitted Diseases Research*. Denver CO. USA, 11–14 July 1999, Abstract No. 487.

26. Obasi, A., Bisecko, S., Gabone, R., Gavyole, A., Grosskurth, H., Hayes, R., *et al.* (1997) Prevention of HIV infection and enhancement of reproductive health among adolescents in rural Tanzania: A community randomized trial. Part 2: Design of the impact evaluation. *12th Meeting of the International Society of Sexually Transmitted Diseases Research.* Seville, Spain, 19–22 October 1997, Abstract No. S44.

27. Cleophas-Frisch, B., Obasi, A., Mshana, G., Wayomi, J., Plummer, M., Rwakatare, M., *et al.* (2001) Use of simulated patients to evaluate youth-friendly reproductive health services in rural Tanzania. *14th Meeting of the International Society of Sexually Transmitted Diseases Research.* Berlin, Germany, 24–27 June 2001, Abstract, p. 209.

28. Plummer, M. (1999) Process Evaluation Report: MEMA kwa Vijana Community and Class Peer Educator Training.

29. Guyon, A., Lugoe, W., and Ferguson, J. (2000) Evaluation Report of HIV/AIDs Peer Education in the MEMA kwa Vijana Project, Mwanza, Tanzania.

30. Airhihenbuwa, C.O. and Obregon, R. (2000) A critical assessment of theories / models used in health communication for HIV/AIDS. *J Health Commun,* **5**(suppl.), 5–15.

31. Buston, K., Wight, D., and Hart, G. (2002) Inside the sex education classroom: the importance of class context in engaging pupils. *Cult Health Sexuality,* **4**, 317–35.

32. Buston, K., Wight, D., and Scott, S. (2002) Implementation of a teacher-delivered sex-education programme: obstacles and facilitating factors. *Health Educ Res,* **17**, 59–72.

33. Obasi, A., Cleophas-Frisch, B., Chima, K.L., Mataba, S., Mmassy, G., and Balira, R., *et al.* (2000) Health worker and head teacher attitudes to the provision of reproductive health education and services to adolescents in rural Mwanza region, Tanzania. *13th International AIDS Conference.* Durban, South Africa, 9–14 July 2000, Abstract No. WePp1334.

34. Woodcock, A., Stenner, K., and Ingham, R. (1992) "All these contraceptives, videos and that…": young people talking about school sex education. *Health Educ Res,* **7**, 517–31.

35. Measor, L., Tiffin, C., and Miller, K. (2000) *Young People's Views on Sex Education: Education, Attitudes and Behaviour.* Routledge Falmer, London.

36. NHS Centre for Reviews & Dissemination. (1997) Preventing and reducing the adverse effects of unintended teenage pregnancies. *Eff Health Care,* **3**, 1–9.

37. Dureya, E.J., Dempsey, T., Okuwumabua, J., and Perry, C. (1988) The Solomon four-group design: an application for health education research. In: Humphrey, J.H. (ed.) *Advances in Health Education: Curr Res,* AMS Press, New York.

38. Petrosino, A., Turpin-Petrosino, C., and Finckenauer, J.O. (2000) *Crime Delinquen,* **46**, 354–79.

39. Plummer, M.L., Wight, D., Ross, D.A., Todd, J., Mosha, F., Obasi, A., *et al.* (1999) Measurement of the impact of a sexual behaviour intervention: an attempt to separate fact from fantasy within an intervention trial. *XIth International Conference on AIDS and STDs in Africa.* Lusaka, Zambia, 12–16 September 1999, Abstract No. 13PT38-14.

Section 3

What happens after a trial is completed?

How can evaluation findings be translated into policy and practice? How can sustainability be achieved? How helpful are systematic reviews and meta-analyses of sexual health interventions?

Chapter 11

Generalizability of trials and implementation of research into practice

Heiner Grosskurth and Lilani Kumaranayake

Introduction

Sexual health intervention trials have no end in themselves. They are conducted to identify effective interventions that will help to reduce health risks in populations. It is therefore important to ensure that trial results are relevant to public health. Results should be generalizable to the entire population at risk (not only the sub sample enrolled for the trial), and as much as possible to populations other than that in which the trial was conducted. The intervention to be tested in the trial should be suitable for large-scale replication. And ultimately the trial should have a tangible influence on health policy.

In this chapter, we look first at factors that determine the extent to which the observed effects in a randomized trial can be generalized to other populations. Some suggestions are proposed to increase generalizability at the design stage. Because populations are heterogeneous, repeat trials in different environments are often required. However, as trials are expensive, the use of computer modelling has been suggested as an alternative to explore likely intervention effects in other populations. The chapter briefly discusses the options and limitations of this strategy.

Translating research results into policy and practice is not straightforward. Various strategies towards achieving this objective are considered, including cost-effectiveness analysis. The last two sections of this chapter are concerned with the practicalities of scaling up an intervention and with aspects of sustainability.

Generalizability

A trial outcome is generalizable if it is valid, *and* if the intervention can be expected to lead to similar results when implemented in other populations.

Validity of trial outcomes

When conducting an intervention trial, we measure the effect of an intervention (e.g. an educational programme for adolescents) on the outcome of interest (e.g. the sexually transmissible infection (STI) prevalence in a population or the incidence of unintended pregnancies). The results will be accepted as valid if we can demonstrate that the observed impact cannot be explained by factors other than the intervention. This requires consideration of methodological criteria that apply to any intervention study. First, we need to choose a sample that is sufficiently large that the play of chance is an unlikely explanation for the observed impact. Second, using stratification and randomization we need to minimize the risk that possible confounding factors may be unevenly distributed between intervention and control groups; and we need to document such factors so that possible imbalances can be adjusted for in the analysis (see Chapter 7). Third, we need to avoid bias, that is a lack of comparability between intervention and control groups. An example illustrates these points: if we want to investigate the impact of periodic presumptive STI treatment among sex workers on the rate of new HIV infections, we need to ensure that (i) the sample size is sufficiently large for a postulated minimum effect to be statistically significant; (ii) the number of sex partners and the level of condom use are documented and shown to be roughly similar in the intervention and control groups both at baseline and at follow-up; and (iii) the two groups are from the same population and exposed to similar risks (e.g. we should not compare the intervention effect among high income sex workers such as call girls with that among low income sex workers such as street based prostitutes).

If these criteria are met, we can conclude that there is a genuine statistical association between intervention and outcome measure. This is not sufficient to prove causality. However, causality can usually be assumed if the sequence of events is unambiguous (i.e. the intervention came first, and the outcome occurred later), and if the link is biologically plausible. Both will usually be the case in prospective studies.

Generalizability to the wider population in which the trial was conducted

Generally, in intervention trials, a sample of the population is recruited and followed over time. Part of the cohort will be exposed to the intervention. Clearly, the observed result refers only to study subjects who participated both at enrolment and at follow-up. The result may therefore not be representative of subjects who were absent at enrolment or declined to participate, or for those who were lost to follow-up. In trials of sexual health interventions, this special form of selection bias is particularly important for the following reasons: (i) it is likely that the more mobile part of the population is at greater risk of unprotected casual sex, (ii) individuals who refuse to participate in the survey may do so because they know that they are at a greater risk and feel embarrassed about it, and (iii) the more mobile part of the population is likely to be less exposed to the intervention. Note that this selection bias occurs in both intervention and control groups, so that it does not invalidate the results of the trial. However, it has a bearing on the generalizability of the results, as the observed impact of a sexual health intervention in the study population is likely to be higher than can be expected in the larger target population.

At the design stage, care can be taken to minimize (although not eliminate) this problem. A thorough information and sensitization campaign can be launched before the start of the trial, with special attention to the more mobile part of the population. During follow-up, repeated attempts should be made to contact participants who were initially absent. However, special efforts to increase the *uptake* of the intervention by the mobile part of the target population should only be made if it is feasible to do so in scaled-up intervention programmes as well. The trial would otherwise lose rather than gain generalizabilty.

Generalizability to other populations

This is an important concern for all intervention trials. Efficacy of a health intervention may vary between populations due to variations in disease appearance and host response. However, generalizability is a particularly important concern in trials of sexual health interventions because populations may differ strongly with respect to STI and HIV epidemiology, sexual behaviour, service uptake, and the local acceptability of particular intervention strategies.

We discuss each of these aspects in turn.

Differences in STI and HIV epidemiology between populations play an important role if the outcome variable of a sexual health intervention trial is a biomedical one, such as HIV incidence or STI prevalence. For example, the effectiveness of STI treatment on HIV transmission will vary depending on the proportion of new HIV infections that can be attributed to concurrent STIs and depending on the prevalence of treatable STIs. Both may be reduced in populations with mature HIV epidemics, because in such epidemics most HIV transmission happens outside high risk groups. As the epidemic matures, more people with HIV have a high viral load, which is associated with a high HIV transmission probability. And in mature epidemics, most genital ulcers are probably caused by herpes-simplex virus-2 infection, which is associated with both increased HIV infectivity and susceptibility, and is hard to treat.

Such epidemiological differences between trial populations may *in part* explain the discrepant results between two STI treatment trials in East Africa.[1] In Mwanza, Tanzania, in a population with low but rising HIV prevalence and high prevalence of bacterial STIs, improved STI services for symptomatic cases were associated with a significant 40 per cent reduction of HIV incidence in the intervention group. However, in Rakai, Uganda in a population with high, stable HIV prevalence and comparatively low prevalence of bacterial STIs, mass treatment of bacterial STI did not change HIV transmission in the intervention group.[1] Similar epidemiological differences are likely to explain the results of the 3-arm trial of Masaka, Uganda, which evaluated a behavioural intervention alone and a behavioural intervention combined with improved STI services. There was no reduction in HIV incidence although condom use had increased in both intervention arms and a reduction in the prevalence of some STIs was observed in the arm with STI services.[2] The importance that the stage of the HIV epidemic has on the effect of HIV prevention strategies has been confirmed by comparative computer modelling.[3] The stage of the epidemic may also have a bearing on behavioural outcomes: where mortality from AIDS is high, the personal experience of AIDS among relatives or neighbours may enhance the effect of behavioural interventions.[4,5]

Differences in sexual behaviour between populations are associated with differences in risk exposure and may therefore influence intervention effectiveness substantially. The underlying determinants of sexual behaviour consist of a wide spectrum of cultural, socio-economic and demographic factors. Examples of these three categories include the cultural acceptability of pre- or extramarital sexual relations, the economic pressure on women to exchange sexual favours for material support, and demographic phenomena such as high concentrations of male migrant workers. A practical example illustrates the influence of these factors over intervention effects. A behavioural intervention among adolescents may greatly reduce risk of infection in a population in which young women have some control over sexual encounters, such as in rural East Africa, but may be much less effective in, for example, rural India, where women marry young and have little or no influence over their sexual life.[6]

Differences in service uptake between populations may be substantial and thus influence intervention effects. For example, STI/HIV intervention projects in rural Africa are often delivered through the systematic provision of training and material support to government health centres and dispensaries. Such interventions have been highly successful in some places, but are likely to achieve little in areas where most people seek care from private providers, as is the case in many areas of Asia.[7,8]

Differences in the acceptability of interventions. Interventions that have been shown to be both acceptable and effective in one population may not work in another. For example, during the 1990s, condom promotion campaigns increased condom use and reduced the risk of infection markedly in urban, but not rural, communities in Tanzania.[9]

These examples suggest that the generalization of trial outcomes across populations remains problematic. Even if an intervention is effective in populations other than the one in which the trial was originally conducted, it is extremely unlikely that the *size* of the effect will be similar to that observed in the trial. Whilst this seems obvious, it is surprising how often the observed size of the impact of a successful intervention is wrongly generalized and applied to all kinds of other conditions. For example, the STI/HIV intervention trial in Mwanza Region showed a reduction in HIV incidence of about 40 per cent in the intervention group in comparison with the control group. The size of the reduction has been uncritically adopted by many as the impact that could be expected anywhere where effective STI case management is introduced.[10] This notion changed only after the contrasting results of the Rakai trial had been published.

Options to deal with limited generalizability

We have seen how limited the generalizability of intervention trials may be. How can we deal with this problem?

First, new public health intervention strategies should be evaluated under conditions that are as representative as possible for the region in which they are located, and for the area where they will be introduced on a larger scale if the trial shows that the intervention is effective. Obviously there is no uniform population, but at least a conscious effort can be made at the design stage of trials to avoid working in special environments, even if these may seem much more convenient from a logistical and financial point of view. For example, an intervention in a rural setting that is based on the promotion and the improvement of reproductive health services can be more easily delivered and evaluated in communities that are accessible by vehicle. However, if most communities are not accessible by road, it would be much more meaningful to conduct the trial in typical communities even though this will substantially increase the duration and costs of the research.

Second, major new public health intervention strategies should undergo *multiple trials* in different populations. These trials should be designed to be complementary, investigating effectiveness in populations with differing epidemiological and behavioural characteristics. It is well accepted that new drugs or vaccines must be evaluated in multiple trials before they are adopted for general use. This principle should apply to new health promotion strategies as well. Unfortunately this principle has not been generally accepted. Critics have claimed that large-scale intervention trials are too expensive and time consuming to justify investing in repeat trials, that too much time would be lost until effective new interventions are widely implemented, and that it would be sufficient to adjust interventions to local conditions and restrict the evaluation to operational aspects. We would argue that promising interventions should not be withheld from populations until repeat trials are completed, but that such trials must be conducted until the body of evidence is sufficiently strong to justify long term allocation of resources.

Third, policy makers should look carefully at the conditions under which a new intervention has been tested, and compare the characteristics of the trial population with that in the region or country where they would like to apply the intervention. They should seek expert advice as to whether the intervention is likely to work under the epidemiological, behavioural and demographic conditions prevailing in those areas.

The use of computer modelling to explore the generalizability of trial results

As discussed above, multiple trials are required before results of one trial can reliably be generalized to other populations. However, randomized controlled intervention trials to evaluate sexual health interventions are often very expensive and time consuming, particularly in developing countries where they may also detract resources away from other important programmes.

Mathematical and stochastic models

To some extent, computer modelling can offer an alternative solution. Computer models can be used to simulate the development of epidemics over time and to predict the impact of health interventions. They use epidemiological, behavioural and demographic background data as inputs to predict outputs such as HIV or STI prevalence or incidence. Interventions can be modelled by manipulating inputs. There are principally two kinds of models which differ with respect to the methodology through which the predicted outputs are generated.[11] Mathematical models use equations to produce these outputs. The equations are designed according to available observational data. Where background data are missing, meaningful assumptions are used instead. In contrast, stochastic models generate a model population to produce the outputs of interest. The model population comprises thousands of virtual individuals who may or may not experience events such as entering a relationship with other individuals, becoming exposed to infection, acquiring an infection, seeking treatment, etc. Events happen according to assigned probabilities that are based on observed data or meaningful assumptions. Because outputs are generated through a combination of chance effects, different model runs will produce somewhat different outputs. Several hundred runs are usually conducted, and outputs averaged to produce a final output.

Expectations and limitations

Computer models are only as reliable as the empirical data used to design them. Unfortunately many important input parameters such as the exact STI/HIV cofactor effects for individual STIs are not yet known. A principle weakness of computer models is that the same outputs can be generated through various different combinations of input assumptions. This makes the construction of a 'true' model difficult.

However, empirical data from well conducted epidemiological studies and intervention trials can help to improve existing models. By combining results from different studies and by experimenting with standardized assumptions for unknown biological parameters (such as transmission probabilities), constraints can be put on the variability of input assumptions, and thus more robust models developed that may even help to predict the likely value for hitherto unknown variables.

It should be emphasized that the methodology is still being developed, and that no models yet exist that would allow the impact of sexual health interventions to be simulated reliably. However, the expectation is that existing models will improve and suitable computer programmes will become widely available. These models will not only be used to obtain context specific estimates of the impact and cost-effectiveness of alternative interventions within a variety of possible scenarios, but will also allow identification of crucial factors that determine (cost-) effectiveness, thereby facilitating health policy decisions.

Cost-effectiveness analysis as a tool to increase the policy relevance of trial results

Objective of cost-effectiveness studies in intervention trials

Randomized controlled trials can show whether or not a proposed intervention is effective. However, before a new intervention is adopted for large-scale use, policy makers will expect information on how costly the intervention is and how cost-effective it is, both in achieving its benefits *per se* and in comparison with other public health interventions. Trial results that are not accompanied by cost-effectiveness data will have more difficulty in being translated into policy, even if the intervention proves to be highly effective. For this reason, collaboration with a health economist should be sought at the start of the planning phase of any intervention trial.

Methodology overview

Cost-effectiveness analysis (CEA) is a method that relates the costs of an intervention to the achieved outcome(s). It will establish effectiveness parameters such as cost per HIV infection averted or operational parameters such cost per condom distributed or per STI patient treated. A key feature of CEA is that it allows the relative efficiency of alternative interventions with the same objective to be assessed through comparison of their costs and outcomes.[12] For example, a particular intervention is more efficient than another if it achieves a specific outcome at less cost, or if it achieves a higher outcome for a given budget. Note that a cost-effective intervention is not necessarily an inexpensive one.

Good CEA requires a well-designed tool for collecting cost data. Cost data comprise capital costs and running costs. Capital costs consist of inputs that have a working life of more than a year, and may include buildings, vehicles, and other durable equipment. Running costs consist of inputs that have a shorter life span and are computed on an annual basis. Running costs may include salaries, fuel and other routine supplies, supervision visits, refresher training, and office running expenses. Data are also collected on start-up costs that can, for example, include the initial training of programme staff or health workers and community sensitization or mobilization campaigns. For the purpose of the analysis, such start-up items are treated as capital costs.

In the cost analysis, capital costs and start-up costs are treated differently from running costs in terms of their allocation over time, because they differ with respect to the time at which the costs are incurred and the time at which they are used or their benefits occur. For example, start-up costs and the purchase of capital items generally occur in the beginning of an intervention programme, but their benefit will be spread across the lifetime of the project. For this reason, such costs are annualized by calculating the annual equivalent costs of these items. Meaningful annual discount rates are applied to reflect the waning value. In contrast, the purchase and the use of items that constitute the running costs of a project will normally occur during the same time intervals, and they are therefore reflected in the current year's cost. Annualized cost of capital and start-up items are added to the running costs of each specific year. The result is averaged to form the total annual cost of the intervention.

Costs associated with routine project monitoring and evaluation should be included in the analysis, because monitoring progress would be part of any good intervention programme. However, costs incurred during the impact evaluation should be excluded, as this is a research activity. This distinction can be difficult if, for example, certain staff members or vehicles are involved in both intervention and outcome evaluation. In such cases costs should be split according to analysis of use. It is not uncommon for the costs of the impact evaluation to far exceed the costs of the intervention. For example, in the Mwanza STI/HIV trial, the annual intervention costs amounted to US$ 59,000[13] only, whilst the annual costs of the overall research programme exceeded US$ 400,000.

The total annual cost of the intervention is then related to units of intervention, resulting in parameters such as 'annual cost per adolescent reached', 'cost per condom distributed', 'cost per STI case treated', 'annual intervention cost per capita of target population' etc. There are detailed guidelines on how to standardize the costing of sexual health interventions,[14] also available as Best Practice Guidelines from UNAIDS or on the internet.[15]

The next step is to relate costs to trial outcomes. For example, where an intervention trial has been conducted to reduce HIV transmission, cost can be expressed as per HIV case prevented. Using standard life tables, the average age at infection in the control group, and the average survival time after infection, it is also possible to calculate the cost per life year saved. If prevented HIV morbidity is included, cost-effectiveness can also be expressed as 'cost per DALY (disability adjusted life year) saved'. This is increasingly used as a standardized approach to measure and compare the cost-effectiveness of different public health interventions.[16,17]

Example: cost-effectiveness analysis of the Mwanza STI intervention

The cost-effectiveness analysis of the Mwanza STI/HIV intervention trial illustrates several of these points.[13] The start-up phase involved building a training hall, repairing health units, refurbishing a reference clinic, training health workers, providing simple equipment to health workers, vehicles for supervisors, and the development of training materials. Total capital expenditures amounted to US$ 37,074. Recurrent expenditures included salaries, car maintenance, fuel, drugs, outstation allowances, and office running costs, and amounted to US$ 81,046 for the two years of intervention. The total cost per STI episode treated was US$ 10.15 and US$ 0.39 was the annual cost per capita of the target population. The latter gives valuable information for health service planners. The intervention prevented 252 cases of HIV infection annually, within the catchment area of the trial, at a cost of US$ 217.62 per prevented infection. Using life expectancies for Tanzanians and for an optimized standard population, intervention costs per DALY saved were estimated at US$ 10.33 and 9.45, respectively. This cost-effectiveness compared favourably with other important public health interventions such as a tuberculosis control programme (US$ 30–50 per DALY saved) or an EPI vaccination programme (US$ 12–17 per DALY saved).[16]

Sensitivity analysis

Cost-effectiveness calculations are usually combined with a sensitivity analysis to explore how cost-effectiveness would differ under different scenarios and to take into account uncertainty in data measurement. These often include higher or lower costs for alternative geographical or administrative settings, higher or lower effectiveness (using confidence intervals around empirical impact results), and higher or lower estimates for any assumptions made in the analysis. Using the above example, the sensitivity analysis for the Mwanza STI/HIV intervention showed that costs per DALY saved ranged from US$ 2.51 to 47.86, depending on whether all positive or all negative parameter ranges were combined. It is reassuring to policy makers that even in the worst case scenario the costs per DALY saved were justifiable and competitive when compared with the clinical management of AIDS patients.

It is important to explore the likely cost-effectiveness of a scaled-up intervention (see below pages 180 and 185). Effectiveness may be somewhat lower in non-trial settings because staff may not be as motivated as those in the trial, or because logistical problems might be more difficult to solve. However, costs, particularly investment costs, will not increase proportionally when an intervention is scaled up. In the example of the Mwanza intervention, it has been possible to extend the intervention from the 25 health units that participated in the trial to more than 150 health units in the same region, without increasing the number of staff or vehicles used for training and supervision.[18] It is estimated that the annual costs per capita of the intervention decreased from US$ 0.39 to 0.25.

Interpretation and generalizability of cost-effectiveness studies

As discussed at the beginning of this chapter, the efficacy of a health intervention may vary between populations and intervention effects cannot be generalized easily without taking account of the specific context of the area of interest. The same is true for cost-effectiveness analyses. Naturally, if outcome measures differ between different settings because of variations in epidemiology, sexual behaviour, and service uptake, *cost*-effectiveness will also vary. However, cost-effectiveness comprises a calculation of both *outcome* and *cost* (see methodology overview below). Therefore any variations in cost between different settings will also influence cost-effectiveness.

Many costs are context specific, because *unit-costs* (e.g. cost per litre of fuel) and the *amount of input* required to achieve the same output (e.g. the distance to be travelled to supervise rural schools) may differ. Other important examples include the salary of teachers or health workers that may differ considerably between different countries. The scale of activity will also influence costs, as the same intervention may be less or more expensive as one moves from a community based intervention to a district-wide intervention. The matter becomes even more difficult and complicated if we attempt to compare the cost-effectiveness of *different* interventions in different settings.

A valid comparison of cost-effectiveness measures between different settings can therefore only be made if sufficient information is provided on all relevant details. It is important to keep this principle in mind when the results of the CEA of a trial are reported. It is insufficient if only average costs per unit of outcome are reported. Instead, all relevant data should be revealed that allow the finding of one study to be translated into the context of another.

Computer models to assess the cost-effectiveness of interventions

A number of useful models are already available to estimate and compare the cost-effectiveness of different reproductive health interventions under different scenarios. These may be useful tools for health policy makers, as long as users are conscious of the underlying assumptions and limitations. Examples include the AVERT model,[19] and *HIVTools*.[20] *HIVTools* consists of (1) guidelines for costing different HIV prevention activities and (2) a set of simulation models that can be used to estimate the impact and the cost-effectiveness of different HIV prevention strategies in different settings. *HIVTools* aims to be flexible and easy to use, designed for policy makers, programme managers, and AIDS service organizations. The package including user guidelines are available from UNAIDS(http://www.unaids.org/publications/documents/economics/index.html#cost_model).

Translating research results into policy and practice

Interaction between research and policy formulation

There has been little research into the interaction between researchers and policy-makers. However, the following observations probably hold true. Researchers often assume that high quality research with conclusive results will automatically influence policy. They tend not to engage in the process of policy formulation itself. This at least partly reflects their preference to stick to their area of expertise, which, in the case of large-scale intervention trials, may include epidemiology, clinical medicine, or anthropology, but not usually health policy. Researchers perceive the process of policy formation as something beyond their control and technical expertise.[10] As a result they are surprised if research results fail to be translated into policy change. The literature about the transfer of research findings into policy entails more failures than successes.[21-25]

In their efforts to spend available resources wisely, policy-makers are subject to similar communication hurdles. Research published in scientific journals is often less penetrable and less relevant than many other influences, such as economic and financial constraints and pressure from lobbying groups. In order to influence policy makers, research needs to make use of strategies that go way beyond ensuring the scientific quality of the research.

Strategies to support the translation of trial results into policy

At the planning stage of a trial, researchers should consider *how* research may have an impact on policy, if a trial shows an intervention to be effective. This should not be an afterthought. Researchers should always be aware of the policy environment, and of factors that may possibly enhance or hinder the translation of results into policy and practice.

Early on, there needs to be frequent dialogue between researchers and policy-makers, so that both become equally conscious of the research question that underlies the trial and its potential implications for policy. Often this dialogue will have to be initiated by researchers who must therefore overcome their natural hesitancy to engage in such talks. Researchers also need to facilitate a process whereby the issue broadly enters public awareness. They should enter into dialogue or even strategic alliances with policy-makers and also with others who have a geographic, academic, development, or political interest in the issue that the trial is addressing.

After completion of the trial, researchers will need to present the results simply and clearly, even if important details are complicated and not easily understood by the non-expert. It is imperative that policy-makers can easily digest the results and can 'sell' them to those whose approval or collaboration is required to effect a policy shift.[10] This is not always easy. Over-simplification must be avoided, as must expectations that cannot be met.

Scaling-up

In a trial, the intervention is typically co-ordinated by a local project management team and implemented by a small number of partner institutions covering a defined area. The key players know each other and are sufficiently motivated to contribute effectively to the project. Problems can usually be solved quickly because communication lines are short. Although the intervention may well be delivered through the existing health care or educational system, key operational functions such as training, supervision, monitoring and administration often remain under direct control of the research team.

Scaling interventions up involves many more players, represents a major managerial and logistic challenge, and sooner or later requires integration into existing hierarchical and logistical systems. This section describes typical problems and pitfalls that occur when interventions are brought to scale. Organizational measures to overcome these problems are also discussed.

Phasing in

The most frequent problem relates to the desire to achieve high coverage within a short time. Policy-makers are under pressure to ensure that an effective intervention will become available to everybody as soon as possible. Pressure is particularly strong in the face of an expanding HIV epidemic. The problem relates not to the original trial, but to the urgency with which policy shifts are expected to occur.

Taking an intervention to scale requires identification and constructive involvement of new stakeholders, transfer of knowledge and skills to many workers, motivation of workers, procurement and delivery of large-scale supplies, and reorganization of responsibilities. These requirements are often interlinked and need to be addressed together in a co-ordinated manner. For example, it is essential to ensure that health workers trained to adopt new treatment guidelines will have access to drugs on completion of training—not long before (as drugs may expire) and not long after (because new knowledge will be forgotten). Because of the complex nature of the task, it is almost inevitable that organizational and managerial mistakes occur. If these occur on a small scale, they can be corrected. However, if upscaling happens quickly, organizational flaws are taken to scale as well, and may even be firmly incorporated into the new structure by the time they are discovered. Rectification will then require major effort and financial resources.

To avoid such problems, scaling-up should be performed stepwise. This applies to both geographical expansion and sectoral extension (e.g. extending an intervention from public health units to government institutions such as the police force, or to private health providers). Each step should include a pilot phase. For example, if an intervention is expanded into other regions or provinces of the country, it should first be piloted in only one district per province, and within that district in only a few sites. If this principle is observed, all managerial authorities in each of the newly included areas will be able to learn from their mistakes, and also from the mistakes of other pilot sites. A precondition for the success of this strategy is acceptance of, and openness about, the problems encountered. In some programmes, this strategy has been successfully used in scaling interventions up.[26]

It is obvious that the stepwise introduction of a new intervention requires time. Depending on the nature of the intervention, a year or more may have to pass until the next step can be taken. It will not always be easy for policy makers to withstand public pressure and accept this comparatively slow pace of progress. However, they should be reassured by the knowledge that this approach leads to a better programme and is also much less costly.

Managerial capacity

The large-scale introduction of a new intervention places a new burden on the management teams that will be responsible for it. The need for additional staff is greatest during the scaling-up phase; it lessens once the new programme is in place everywhere and a steady state has been reached. Unfortunately, the additional burden is often placed on top of existing programmes without providing additional managerial capacity. This is the other major problem that can turn a good new intervention programme into an ailing or failing investment.

The solution lies in the allocation of additional competent full-time staff at all levels involved in the new programme. At central level, for example, within the ministry of health, a task force or central support unit is usually required. For example, when national STI control programmes were introduced in many developing countries, they were placed within existing national AIDS control programmes. Such a task force would normally have a programme manager, and should include officers for training, supervision, and operational monitoring, logistics, and administration. At lower management levels, task forces would have fewer members, or may comprise only one person. However, it is important that these officers are also fully dedicated to the programme and have no other duties. To avoid adverse effects of the new programme on existing activities, regular liaison and co-ordination is required with the managerial units that are responsible for other programmes, again at all levels.

Logistics

During intervention trials, the supply of health education materials, medicines, condoms, or other consumables is under the control of the intervention manager, but this is not usually possible for large-scale programmes. For example, the provision of trial drugs would normally be the responsibility of the central medical store or equivalent unit, rather than the task force. This dissociation of previously joint functions is the third important potential cause of unsuccessful scaling-up. For example, the Mwanza STI control programme was expanded stepwise to comparison communities and then to most other health units of the region and to selected communities in neighbouring regions. Supplies were provided reliably to peripheral health units through the same non-governmental organization that implemented the original trial. About two years after trial, the intervention was also introduced in many other regions of the country. At that time, provision of drugs was transferred to the national programme. Despite adequate funding, and the managers' best efforts, the supply of drugs soon became erratic and health units repeatedly ran out of drugs for long periods, resulting in great frustration among peripheral health workers and a substantial decline in the quality of the programme.

Such unfortunate situations could be avoided by temporarily creating contingency supplies at different levels that function like a buffer in case of breakdown of supplies. These buffer stocks should be in place before integration into routine structures begins, and they should remain under the direct control of the central support unit. The introduction of buffer stocks does not imply creating a parallel system, but is a temporary measure to bridge the period of irregular supplies that will almost inevitably occur during logistical transfer from a centralized to an integrated system. The central support unit will need to monitor the flow of supplies to and from buffer stocks so that stocks do not expire. Again, this is easier to achieve if the intervention is scaled up stepwise.

Human resources

Scaling up an intervention means motivating, training, and intensively supporting a large group of competent peripheral implementers. This can be a major operational task.

Motivation

Whilst the senior staff of the original trial intervention will naturally perceive a new effective intervention as highly important, for peripheral workers it may simply mean extra work. The fact that the trial results were impressive is not usually sufficient to create enthusiasm. But peripheral workers, whether teachers, physicians, medical assistants, or community workers, are the most important stakeholders to the successful scaling-up of a new programme. So what is in for them? Financial incentives will not usually be feasible in resource poor countries. And since the work will eventually have to become part of routine duties, it is generally unwise to offer financial incentives to non-research staff during intervention trials.

However, the conditions that need to be met for successful scaling-up are similar to those required for successful conduct of the trial. In most intervention trials these conditions are met in a number of ways: by holding meetings to motivate the community and foster a positive attitude towards the new service; by informing those who implement the intervention about the importance of the intervention to the health of their community; by holding training sessions; by visiting staff and monitoring their activities which thereby reinforces the importance of their work. All this creates a conducive environment that convinces peripheral workers that the new activity is important and gives workers a chance to escape their usual routine for a short time and learn something new.

It is important to try to create the same conditions when scaling-up an intervention. Although it will not be possible to hold meetings with all village authorities, it is possible to sensitize the public to the new intervention through the media, government information channels, or in other ways. Peripheral workers should not just be instructed to perform the new activities (as is so often the case), but should be informed about the importance of the work and trained in a stimulating and effective way.

Training

A typical misconception is that a short series of training courses will suffice and that staff who have attended a seminar or course will put a new intervention into practice when told to do so. However, this is rarely the case. Whilst staff may have understood and accepted a new intervention strategy intellectually, they often hesitate to implement it, particularly if the new strategy involves major emotional effort or adopting unfamiliar principles. For example, many doctors in developing countries claim to use the syndromic strategy for STI case management, but have difficulty in following it in practice because it seems to deviate from the principle of providing treatment on the base of a precise diagnosis.[27] Similarly, although life skills including AIDS prevention education have been officially introduced as a subject into the curricula of schools in many countries, few of the trained teachers have actually implemented these curricula because they feel uncomfortable with the topic.

How can this dilemma be solved? Taking the example of a school based educational intervention, formal training courses have to be followed up by a phase of in-service training whereby staff implement what they have learned with the support of an experienced trainer. Trainers from the original trial intervention team should join the central support unit temporarily for this purpose. Once the intervention is in place in a small number of pilot schools, their experience can be used to train and support others. During this snowballing process, the role of central support unit staff will change from training to supervision and programme monitoring. Although this approach is time consuming, it is essential for effective large-scale implementation.

Support supervision

Even after training, regular supervision will be needed during routine programme implementation to reassure staff, provide feedback, and solve problems. This is essentially the way to ensure the quality of the programme. Once implementation is in full swing and staff become self-reliant, the intensity of supervision can be reduced stepwise. Supervision should be a supportive and creative activity rather than a strategy to maintain discipline. To emphasize this aspect, the term 'supervision' is increasingly being replaced by 'support supervision'. The importance of support supervision for a new intervention programme cannot be over-emphasized: staff should only be trained if their supervision is guaranteed, and the capacity of the programme to provide in-service training and support supervision is the time limiting factor in the process of scaling-up.

Costs of scaling-up: the importance of infrastructural limits

When scaling up an intervention, the time-frame and costs or altering inputs and increasing capacity need careful consideration. Some inputs can be increased more easily than others. For example, variable inputs, such as drugs and other supplies, can be adjusted to match the number of people to be reached by the scaled-up intervention. In contrast, fixed inputs (often described as infrastructure), such as the number of health facilities, are difficult to adjust in the short-term. Semi-fixed items are a composite of these two categories, consisting of capital items such as vehicles and other equipment which normally do not vary, and whose expected life-time is more than one year.

Initially, as coverage is expanded, average programme costs per unit of measurement (e.g. per adolescent reached) are likely to decrease, whilst total costs expand. However, beyond a certain level of coverage (e.g. 60 per cent), a substantial increase in infrastructure may be needed and there may be a large jump or discontinuity in average costs before coverage can be increased further. Examples include building additional peripheral health units, or an increase in the number of trained teachers, or expansion of the fleet of vehicles used to deliver the intervention. For practical purposes, this threshold can be thought of as the *limit* to scaling-up given *current* levels of capacity. In the long-run, a substantial increase in infrastructure may be needed in order to increase coverage.[28]

Analysis and consideration of stakeholders

Before a programme is taken to scale, a thorough situation analysis[29] and stakeholder analysis should be undertaken.[30] The results should be used to develop a strategy that paves the way for large-scale introduction of the intervention. Stakeholders are those who can be expected to gain or lose as a result of the programme. Whilst the target group is often referred to as 'primary stakeholders', it is the secondary stakeholders on whom the success of the intervention depends. Secondary stakeholders are, for example, the staff that manage a disease control programme. There may be many different groups of secondary stakeholders.

Individuals who lose power or benefits because of the programme are not always obvious. However, they may be influential and could potentially threaten the programme. Unless such stakeholders have been identified, programme implementers may suddenly encounter obstacles whose origin they do not understand. It is therefore of paramount importance to identify major stakeholders during the initial situational analysis, understand their concerns and, if they pose a genuine threat, to plan the programme in such a way that their concerns can be accommodated or circumvented.

For example, in a programme to control HIV infection and other STI among bar girls in a large African city, a drop-in centre was established where women were offered health education, condoms, and syndromic STI case management. Women were invited to come for regular check ups and were encouraged to work together to enforce '100 per cent condom use'. Initially, bar owners were fiercely opposed to the programme on grounds that customers would be unwilling to use condoms or might stay away altogether for fear that the women had AIDS. The problem was overcome once bar owners were invited to a series of short seminars in which the rationale of the programme was discussed and fears addressed. The programme also met clandestine opposition from medical practitioners who provided most of the STI treatment in the area. One of these practitioners was well connected to higher authorities in the municipality, and the programme was suddenly confronted with administrative complaints which took a while to resolve. This problem might have been avoided, had key practitioners been invited to participate in the programme in some way, perhaps by providing training on effective STI treatment or becoming experts to whom more complicated cases could be referred.

Achieving sustainability

The sustainability of a new intervention should be considered at the planning stage of the trial. It is ethically questionable to evaluate an intervention that cannot be sustained in the trial population or replicated on a large scale elsewhere in the country. There are a number of aspects to sustainability, some of which are controversial.

Financial sustainability

This is often thought to be the most important issue. The question typically asked is: can the health system afford to implement the intervention on a large scale if it is shown to be effective? Or can the country ever be expected to keep the intervention going without external funding? Interestingly, in many cases, the answer is neither simple nor static. The debate about provision of anti-retroviral therapy to AIDS patients in developing countries is a good example of how controversial this issue is and how quickly the situation can change. By the end of the 1990s, most people thought that antiretroviral therapy was simply not an option for resource poor countries in the foreseeable future. We are now in the middle of developments which challenge this conviction.

There are countries where the question of financial sustainability of a public health intervention is almost meaningless because their public sector has been heavily subsidized for decades. Here, the appropriate question is not simply how much an intervention costs, but whether it is sufficiently cost-effective and important to compete for existing resources or to attract additional funding. In this situation, other aspects of sustainability become more important: managerial feasibility, cultural and political acceptability and affordability at the level of the target population.

Sustainability can be thought of on two interrelated levels. Sustainability usually implies lessening the reliance on external resources, which in many countries means achieving an appropriate balance between national government and donor resources. This is referred to as the capacity for continuity. At a second level, sustainability is concerned with the ability of the programme to secure sufficient resources locally (from national government and private sources) and to use the resources effectively and efficiently. This is referred to as financial sustainability.[31]

Managerial feasibility

This aspect addresses important questions such as; can sufficient highly skilled and motivated staff be made available to take on the new task? Does this require removing staff from other programmes that are running well, and if so how would those programmes suffer?

Cultural acceptability

Even when interventions are conceptually clear and the evidence for their effectiveness is convincing, implementation may be patchy if the interventions are not culturally acceptable in specific situations. For example, research has demonstrated that 100 per cent condom use by sex workers in Thailand drastically reduced the incidence of new HIV infections and STIs in this group and among their clients.[32] However, in some parts of India, sex workers do not have the power to even suggest condom use with their regular partners who control the sex trade and who themselves are often highly promiscuous.[33] It is very difficult to mount a meaningful and sustainable intervention under these circumstances. Another example is the total failure of a well equipped, hospital-based STI clinic in an African city to attract female sex workers for STI treatment. This was because the sex workers feared that they would lose their job as bar girls or would lose clients, if word spread that they attended this clinic. A completely different intervention had to be established to overcome this problem (E Matasha, personal communication).

Affordability for the target population

Much attention has been given to the financial affordability and sustainability of interventions from the provider perspective. The perspective of the target population is at least as important. For example, an intervention that requires patients to undergo STI testing and return some days later for laboratory results and treatment implies that people can afford to be absent from their normal work for at least two mornings. If, as commonly, this is not the case, the intervention will not be feasible.

Conclusion

This chapter has considered a wide range of issues relating to the generalizability of effective interventions. Many of these issues require careful discussion or negotiation with stakeholders at the planning stage of the trial. They should not become afterthoughts. Cost-effective analysis, feasibility—whether financial, managerial, or cultural—and scaling-up in a phased fashion, are key determinants of the successful and sustainable implementation of sexual health interventions on a large scale.

Acknowledgement

We thank Richard Hayes for his contribution to this chapter.

References

1. Grosskurth, H., Gray, R., Hayes, R., Mabey, D., and Wawer, M. (2000) Control of sexually transmitted diseases for HIV-1 prevention: understanding the implications of the Mwanza and Rakai trials. *Lancet*, **355**, 1981–7.

2. **Kamali, A.** (2001) A community randomized trial of sexual behaviour and syndromic management interventions on HIV transmission in rural Uganda. Presentation at a WHO *Consultation Meeting on STI Case Management.*

3. **Korenromp, E.L., Van Vliet, C., Grosskurth, H., Gavyole, A., Van der Ploeg, C.P.B., Fransen, L., Hayes, R.J., and Habbema, D.** (2000) Model-based evaluation of single-round mass treatment of sexually transmitted diseases for HIV control in a rural African population. *AIDS*, **14**, 573–93.

4. **Kilian, A., Gregson, S., Ndyanabangi, B.,** *et al.* (1999) Reductions in risk behaviour provide the most consistent explanation for declining HIV-1 prevalence in Uganda. *AIDS*, **13**, 391–8.

5. **Konde-Lule, J., Musagara, M., and Musgrave, S.** (1993) Focus group interviews about AIDS in Rakai district of Uganda. *Soc Sci Med*, **37**, 679–84.

6. **Jejeebhoy, S.** (1996) Adolescent sexual and reproductive behaviour. A review of the evidence from India. *International Centre for Research on Women.* Washington, Report No.: ICRW Working Paper No. 3.

7. **Benjarattanaporn, P., Lindan, C.P., Mills, S.,** *et al.* (1997) Men with sexually transmitted diseases in Bangkok: where they go for treatment and why? *AIDS*, **11**(Suppl. 1), S87–S95.

8. **Nandan, D., Gupta, V.K., Dabral, S.B., Misra, S.K., Gupta, S.C., Prakash, B., and Nilaratan, B.** (1999) Role of traditional healers and indigenous medical practitioners in health care. *Indian J Public Health*, **23**, 2.

9. **Munguti, K., Grosskurth, H., Newell, J., Senkoro, K., Mosha, F., Todd, J., Mayaud, P., Gavyole, A., Quigley, M., and Hayes, R.** (1997) Patterns of sexual behaviour in a rural population in north-western Tanzania. *Soc Sci Med*, **44**, 1553–661.

10. **Philpott, A., Maher, D., and Grosskurth, H.** (2002) Translating HIV/AIDS research findings into policy: lessons from a case study of 'the mwanza trial'. *Health Policy Plan*, **2**, 196–201.

11. **Boily, M.-C. and Masse, B.** (1997) Mathematical models of disease transmission: a previous tool of the study of sexually transmitted diseases. *Can J Public Health Med*, **88**, 255–65.

12. **Creese, A. and Parker, D.** (1994) *Cost Analysis in Primary Health Care: A Training Manual for Programme Managers.* WHO, Geneva.

13. **Gilson, L., Mkanje, R., Grosskurth, H., Mosha, F., Picard, J., Gavyole, A., Todd, J., Mayaud, P., Swai, R., Fransen, L., Mabey, D., Mills, A., and Hayes, R.** (1997) Cost-effectiveness of improved treatment services for sexually transmitted diseases in preventing HIV-1 infection in Mwanza region, Tanzania. *Lancet*, **350**, 1805–9.

14. **Janowitz, B. and Bratt, J.H.** (1994) Methods for costing family planning services. United Nations Population Fund and Family Health International.

15. **Kumaranayake, L., Pepperall, J., Goodman, H., Mills, A., and Walker D.** (2000) Costing guidelines for HIV/AIDS prevention strategies. *UNAIDS Best Practice Collection—Key Materials.* Also http://www.unaids.org/highbrand/document/economics/index.html.

16. **World Bank.** (1993) *World Development Report 1993: Investing in Health.* Oxford University, New York.

17. **Murray, C.** (1994) Quantifying the burden of disease: the technical basis for disability-adjusted life years. *Bull WHO*, **72**, 429–45.

18. Attawell, K. and Grosskurth, H. (1999) From knowledge to practice: STI control and HIV prevention. Official Publications of the European Communities.

19. Rehle, T., *et al.* (1998) AVERT: a user-friendly model to estimate the impact of HIV/sexually transmitted disease prevention interventions on HIV transmission. Also at Http://Www.Iaen.Org/Models/Avert/Index.Htm. AIDS **12**(suppl. 2), S27–S35.

20. Watts, C., Kumaranayake, L., Vickerman, P., and Terris-Prestholt, F. (2001) HIVTools: a cost-effectiveness toolkit for prevention. *HIVTools.* Research Working Paper, LSHTM.

21. Appleby, J., Walschee, K., and Ham, C. (1995) *Acting on the Evidence.* Health Service Management Centre, Birmingham.

22. Crosswaite, C. and Curtice, L. (1994) Dissemination research results—the challenge of bridging the gap between health research and health action. *Health Promot Int*, **9**(4), 289–97.

23. Frenk, J. (1992) Balancing relevance and excellence: organizational responses to link research with decision making. *Soc Sci Med*, **35**(11), 1397–401.

24. Garner, P., Kale, R., Dickson, R., Dans, T., and Salinas, R. (1998) Getting research findings into practice: implementing research findings in developing countries. *Br Med J*, **317**, 531–5.

25. King, L., Hawe, P., and Wise, M. (1998) Making dissemination a two way process. *Health Promot Int*, **13**(3), 237–43.

26. Binswanger, H.P. (2000) Scaling up HIV/AIDS programs to national coverage. *Science*, **288**, 2173–5.

27. Kumar, B., Handa, S., and Dawn, G. (1995) Syndromic management of genital ulcer disease—a critical appraisal. *Genitourin Med*, **71**, 197.

28. Kumaranayake, L., Kurowski, C., and Conteh, L. (2001) Costs of scaling-up priority-health interventions for low-income countries. Discussion Paper No. 19, Working Group 5, *Commission on Macroeconomics and Health.* WHO, Geneva. Also http://www.cmhealth.org.

29. Green, A. (1999) *Introduction to Health Planning in Developing Countries* (2nd edition) Oxford University Press, Oxford.

30. Varvasovsky, Z. and Brugha, R. (2000) How to do a stakeholder analysis. *Health Policy Plann*, **15**(3), 338–45.

31. La Fond, A. (1995) *Sustaining Primary Health Care.* Earthscan Publications, London.

32. Hanenberg, R.S., Rojanapithayakorn, W., Kunasol, P., and Sokal, D.C. (1994) Impact of Thailand's HIV-control programme as indicated by the decline of sexually transmitted diseases. *Lancet*, **344**, 243.

33. Nag, M. (2002) *Sexual Behaviour and AIDS in India.* Vikas Publishing, New Delhi.

Chapter 12

The limits of generalizability: community-based sexual health interventions among gay men

Graham Hart and Jonathan Elford

Introduction

In this chapter we use two controlled trials of peer-led interventions as case studies to illustrate some of the problems of generalizing or transferring sexual health interventions from one developed country to another. We begin with the rationale for peer-led community interventions and the success of this approach with gay men in the United States. We then describe attempts to transfer such interventions to the United Kingdom, and consider the implications of this experience.

Peer-led interventions in HIV prevention

During the 1990s there was much interest in the potential of community-based interventions for HIV prevention among gay men, spurred on by what was considered to be the success of such programmes in the United States.[1–3] Peer education was particularly appealing on a number of levels. *Intellectually* it was supported by social theory concerning the 'diffusion of innovations';[4] *intuitively* it made sense since we are most likely to respond to people we know and respect; *financially* it seemed to offer a low cost intervention due to reliance on unpaid volunteers; and *emotionally* it appealed to the altruism of individuals and the community spirit of a group already stigmatized by HIV/AIDS.[5]

Jeffrey Kelly and his colleagues were the first to report on peer-led HIV prevention among gay men. They examined the impact of peer education on the sexual risk behaviour of men attending gay bars in small mid-western towns in the United States.[6,7] Popular men, identified by people working in the bars, were recruited as peer educators to endorse changes in both sexual behaviour and sexual norms. After training, the peer educators were asked to talk to a minimum of 10 other gay men in the bars about HIV risk reduction. The intervention was introduced into one city while two other cities served as controls.[6] Surveys were conducted among gay men using the bars in all three cities before and after the intervention. In the intervention city, the proportion of men who engaged in unprotected anal intercourse decreased by about one third following the intervention, whereas no change was observed among men using bars in the control cities. The authors later evaluated this peer education intervention elsewhere in the United States and found once again that while gay men in intervention bars reported a reduction in high risk sexual behaviour, no such change was reported by the control communities.[1]

Other researchers in the United States took up the challenge of introducing community-based interventions in which peer-educators played a major part. In a trial evaluating the impact of peer education among young gay men living in Eugene (Oregon) and Santa Barbara (California), there was also a significant reduction in the frequency of unprotected anal intercourse with both regular and casual partners following the intervention.[2] One community (Eugene) was initially randomized to the intervention, which included peer education while the other (Santa Barbara) was randomized to the control, where there was no targeted HIV prevention programme for young gay men at the time. Following the intervention in Eugene, the proportion of men engaging in unprotected anal sex decreased by 27 per cent, including a 45 per cent reduction for non-primary partners, and a 24 per cent reduction for primary partners. There were no significant changes in Santa Barbara during the same time period. The prevention programme was then delivered in Santa Barbara, California, where similar reductions in risk behaviour were observed.[3]

At a theoretical level, these peer education programmes draw on a diffusion of innovation model,[4] whereby popular opinion leaders engage in conversation with gay men to promote and endorse HIV risk reduction. According to this model, behaviour change is initially propelled by 'early adopters' or trendsetters, who are often popular, well-regarded individuals. They then communicate this change to other people who adopt it in turn, and gradually the change in behaviour diffuses through the population. The aim of the intervention is to make initial contact with a proportion of the community—not everyone needs direct early contact to be affected. According to the model, the intervention will in time have a community-wide impact through a ripple-like social transmission or diffusion of new ideas. Thus the innovation will, through persuasion and example, permeate the community as a whole and become a community norm. The model is considered to be well suited to community-level HIV prevention campaigns that encourage the adoption of risk reduction behaviour. Such campaigns typically aim for the initiation, diffusion, and long-term maintenance of behaviour change.[8]

In 1996, Janet Holland and others undertook a systematic review of health promotion interventions among gay men.[9] They found that few interventions in this area had been well evaluated, but judged Jeffrey Kelly's studies in the United States to be methodologically sound and peer education to be promising. Together with Susan Kegeles' subsequent work,[2,3] this led to an expectation that community-based interventions using local opinion-leaders could produce significant and demonstrable reductions in HIV-related sexual behaviour.

Encouraging as the North American studies are, it cannot be assumed that they are directly transferable from the United States to other countries, from small towns to large metropolitan areas, or between areas at different stages in the HIV epidemic. Consequently, Holland *et al.*[9] recommended that interventions using peer educators be formulated and evaluated in the United Kingdom in methodologically sound trials. Controversially, one of the criteria for methodological soundness was that the intervention should be evaluated by means of a *randomized controlled trial*, as had been the case in Kelly's studies.

We therefore conducted two community-based trials, one in Scotland (the Gay Men's Task Force), the other in London (the 4 Gym Study) to determine whether it was possible to transfer this model of peer education from the United States to the United Kingdom with the same degree of success. In this chapter, we reflect on our findings, and explore some of the realities of the organization, delivery, and transferability of peer education programmes.

The Gay Men's Task Force

The primary aims of the Gay Men's Task Force (GMTF) were to reduce the incidence of unprotected anal intercourse with casual partners among gay men in Glasgow by 20 per cent, and to increase their uptake of sexual health services, particularly, hepatitis B vaccination.[10] The intervention group comprised gay men using bars in Glasgow, while the control group was made up of gay men using bars in Edinburgh. Since there is very little movement of men between the gay scenes of Glasgow and Edinburgh the two cities provided relatively discrete environments where the intervention could be introduced into one without affecting ('contaminating') the other.[10] The design of the evaluation included baseline measures of sexual behaviour and service use among gay men visiting bars in Glasgow and Edinburgh[11], the provision of a new intervention in Glasgow (but not Edinburgh), and then a post-intervention survey six months later in both cities to compare any reported changes in outcomes.

The GMTF was an inter-agency collaboration consisting of three elements: peer-led sexual health promotion conducted on the commercial gay scene; gay-specific genitourinary medicine (GUM) services in both hospital and gay community settings; and a free-phone 'hotline' providing sexual health information and details of local sexual health services. The free-phone hotline was the least successful element of the intervention. Since only 25 per cent ($n = 45$) of calls in the first six months were genuine, the hotline was suspended, while the other two parts of the GMTF continued for nine months in total.

The 42 peer educators (38 men and 4 women) were recruited from a variety of sources, including the commercial gay scene and voluntary HIV-related organizations.[10,12] They received two days of training and continued support throughout the intervention. Training involved communication skills, role play on approaching men, and specified message delivery. They distributed sexual health promotion materials within bars, then engaged in focused interactions with men in relation to a variety of sexual health issues (primarily Hepatitis B, HIV antibody testing, and HIV risks within relationships). The peer educators recorded a total of 1484 interactions, of an average duration of 10 min, throughout the intervention period.

The 4 gym project

In the North American studies[1] men using bars in one town rarely, if ever, went to bars in any other town. This was also the case in Scotland, so that mixing of patrons between the intervention and control cities (or contamination) was effectively avoided. In London, by contrast, it would be difficult to achieve such distinct intervention and control groups because there is considerable movement of patrons between gay bars. Therefore, we chose to evaluate a peer-led HIV prevention programme among gay men who use *gyms* in central London.[13] Within central London five gyms were identified with a large or exclusively gay membership. Because people often take out a 12 month subscription, they tend to go regularly to one gym only.[14] Thus these gyms provided relatively discrete environments with low risk of contamination during a controlled trial.

Gym managers were asked to identify potential peer educators according to defined criteria. People selected were to be popular, well-known, good communicators and belong to a social network based on, for example, age, ethnicity or time of day they used the gym. Those who expressed interest in the project were invited to a one day training session which covered basic facts and misconceptions about HIV infection; new treatments; strategies for risk reduction; HIV testing; use and misuse of steroids. Communication skills played a large part with activities throughout the day to encourage the peer educators to listen, reflect, summarize and impart knowledge.[13] After training, peer educators ($n = 27$) were asked to talk to at least 20 gay men in their gym over the next five months about HIV risk reduction, focusing on sexual behaviour, HIV testing, relationships, new therapies and the use of steroids. As an incentive, peer educators were offered a payment equivalent to 3 month's gym membership (approximately £100) in return for working the full intervention period.

The primary aims of the 4 gym project were to reduce the proportion of men reporting UAI with a partner of unknown HIV status by one-third and to increase the percentage of men who had ever been tested for HIV from 65 per cent to 75 per cent.[13] Gay men using the gyms were surveyed at baseline and then at 6, 12 and 18 months, in a series of cross-sectional follow up surveys, to monitor changes in outcome.

In both studies, follow-up could include men who happened to be in the bars or gyms at that time, regardless of whether they had been contacted by a peer educator during the intervention. According to the theory of "diffusion of innovation", the intervention should be able to achieve an effect beyond those men approached directly by the peer educators.

Findings

Both studies came up with the same finding—the peer education programmes had no significant impact on sexual risk behaviour, HIV testing or service uptake at a community level.

Gay Men's Task Force

In Glasgow, the only significant temporal change was an increase in the proportion of men reporting Hepatitis B vaccination (49.7% vs 43.8%, $\chi^2 = 8.792$, $p = 0.003$).[15] No significant changes over time were observed for men in Edinburgh. There was also a non-significant temporal change in reported levels of unprotected anal intercourse with casual partners, with a reduction in the proportion of Glasgow men reporting unprotected anal intercourse with at least one casual partner in the previous year and an increase in unprotected anal intercourse with at least one casual partner amongst men in Edinburgh. However, there was no significant interaction between location (Glasgow vs Edinburgh) and time (baseline vs follow-up) that could be attributed to the GMTF intervention.

Nearly a third (32%) of men surveyed in Glasgow post-intervention reported contact with a peer educator, and more either recognized the GMTF symbol (42%) or could correctly specify the words that constitute the acronym (36%).[16] In an "on-treatment" analysis, comparing men who reported contact with a peer educator with other men in Glasgow who reported no contact, we were able to show an intervention effect on sexual behaviour and sexual health service use. However, as with any on-treatment analysis, the findings are subject to bias. In particular, this analysis may simply compare a motivated group of men—who are more likely to speak to a peer educator and more likely to change their sexual behaviour regardless of the peer educator—with a less motivated group. Either way, our qualitative and process evaluations support the finding that the intervention had no significant impact on sexual behaviour at a community level.[17] The peer educators found it difficult to discuss sexual behaviours such as unprotected anal intercourse and emotional issues such as relationships with partners.

4 gym project

The peer-led intervention among gay men using central London gyms had no significant impact on their risk behaviour.[14] Overall the proportion of men reporting high risk sexual behaviour (unprotected anal intercourse with a person of unknown HIV status) varied little between baseline (13.9%) and 18 month follow-up (14.2%, $p = 0.5$), while the percentage of men ever-tested for HIV increased from 73.0 per cent to 79.6 per cent ($p = 0.002$). However, there were no significant differences between intervention and control gyms in the magnitude of change for either outcome. In other words, there was no significant interaction between location (intervention vs control) and time (baseline vs follow-up) ($p >= 0.1$). Why not? Why did this peer-led approach, shown to be effective in the United States, fail to have any significant impact on the risk behaviours of gay men in this London study? What does this tell us about transferability?

Process evaluation, based on interviews with peer educators, the health promotion team and gym managers throws light on this question.[18] Attrition was an important factor. Only one-in-five people initially approached served as peer educators throughout the project, thus limiting the potential for diffusion. Of the 144 potential peer educators identified by gym managers, half (78) expressed an interest in joining the project, a third (42) actually attended a training day while one-fifth (27) worked as peer educators throughout the intervention period. There were three main factors that accounted for this high rate of attrition: lack of time, lack of interest, and lack of confidence.

Those who did go on to work as peer educators reported barriers to communication within the gym, which limited the extent to which diffusion could occur. When interviewed, they said that discussing sex was difficult and that it was hard to approach complete strangers. The peer educators offered a number of useful insights into the difficulties they experienced. Some thought that approaching a stranger in London gyms with a large gay clientele may be interpreted as a sexual advance; others felt that a US model of health promotion, developed in small towns, did not transfer directly to gyms in London; that the intervention may work better in small towns than big cities; and that the intervention period was not long enough to establish a rapport with gym members. These findings raise the question as to whether the gyms constituted true communities: diffusion requires certain structural features to be in place, notably respect for 'early adopters' and interconnectedness of social networks. This emphasises the importance of pre-study formative research which, in this case, was not possible because of limited resources.

The fact that the peer educators found it difficult to hold conversations with gay men in the gyms further limited the extent to which diffusion occurred, which was reflected in the outcome evaluation.[14] Although half the gay men surveyed in the gyms were aware that peer educators had been working in their gyms, only three per cent said they had spoken to a peer educator during the intervention period. Consequently the critical mass required for diffusion was not established. Rather than peer education not working, it simply did not occur. This explains why the intervention had no significant impact on gay men's risk behaviours. Barriers to effective peer education may have been specific to the gym environment. But the obstacles to communication may also have reflected differences between small towns and large cities as well as cultural differences between the UK and US gay men in their interaction with peers.

The Gay Men's HIV Prevention Team found that recruiting, training and supporting peer educators took much more time than they had originally expected.[18] On average the programme required 16.4 hours per week of a health promotion worker's time over 18 months. This is the equivalent of one person spending nearly 2.5 days a week on the project. Almost half the time was spent training and a further third supporting the peer educators.

Implications

In both London and Glasgow we found that a model of peer education, shown to be effective in the United States, had no significant impact on gay men's sexual risk behaviour at a community level.[19] In London, lack of diffusion seemed to account for this finding since only three per cent of men said they had spoken to a peer educator. Peer education simply did not happen. However, in Glasgow a third of gay men surveyed six months post-intervention said they had spoken to a peer educator yet still there was no impact on any outcome at a community level. This indicates that even where peer educators are able to make substantial contact with their target community, diffusion of innovation may not necessarily occur.

In London, we recommended that peer education should not continue in the gyms since there was no evidence that it had any significant impact on gay men's risk behaviours. Our process evaluation also suggested that this *particular* model of peer education was unlikely to succeed in London gay bars either, a conclusion strengthened by the findings from the Glasgow study. The gym managers in London were disappointed by these findings. They saw their gyms as a place for promoting health and fitness among their entire membership and not simply a venue for body building. Consequently, the peer education programme had integrated well with their holistic view of health promotion. Although the gym environment may be less conducive to peer education than originally thought, it may lend itself to other projects led directly by gym staff or the health promotion team. One example is an exercise programme currently run by some of the gyms for people with HIV infection with a focus on overall health as well as fitness.

An important finding from the process evaluation in London is that peer education is not a "cheap option". While peer educators received only a modest payment, the costs to the health promotion team of recruiting, training, and supporting the peer educators were substantial.

In Glasgow it appears that rather than educating their peers, and this message being taken on board both by individuals with whom they had contact and then by the community as a whole, the 'peer educators' actually served as indigenous health outreach workers, facilitating access to sexual health services. This was not 'diffusion of innovation' but advertising, increasing the take-up of available service provision among those with whom direct contact was made. To a health service lacking a significant evidence base on which to plan health promotion services, this has proved useful. Lothian Health Board was not required, on the basis of this research, to start using peer educators to influence community norms, but could encourage Edinburgh-based Gay Men's Health to undertake bar-based work advertising clinical services. Greater Glasgow Health Board saw significant increases in patient numbers as a result of the intervention, and a new 'peer education' programme based in the gay-men specific GUM clinic is being introduced to bars because of the finding that the use of bar-based health outreach workers can increase the number and range of gay men accessing its sexual health services.

Conclusion

In the introduction, we noted that peer education appealed at a number of levels: intellectual, intuitive, financial, and emotional. Our research has demanded that we reconsider each of these. Intellectually, while peer education is supported by social theory, it may not be applicable in all settings. Intuitively, we are still most likely to respond to people we know and respect, but in practical terms it is difficult to recruit, train and support sufficient numbers of these people to be effective at a community level in discussing sex and sexuality. Financially, peer education is not necessarily a cheap option, although if it were to prove effective in changing sexual behaviour and preventing HIV transmission the human and economic costs saved would be considerable. Emotionally, in large cities with established commercial gay scenes and relatively sophisticated and well informed gay men, we may have to reconsider how far we can rely on individuals to be 'product champions', particularly of well established (rather than novel) ideas such as safe sex.

Our research suggests that a model of peer education found to be successful in small US towns in the early 1990s may not transfer to large metropolitan areas in the United Kingdom at the end of that decade—a decade in which highly active antiretroviral treatments were developed and made widely available in developed countries. However, we should not dismiss the possibility that peer education could succeed in small towns in the United Kingdom, similar to the small towns in the United States where the model was first evaluated. Effective behavioural interventions to reduce the risk of HIV infection among gay men are still urgently needed. However, such interventions should undergo piloting or other preliminary assessment before evaluation on a larger scale.

References

1. Kelly, J.A., Murphy, D.A., Sikkema, K.J., McAuliffe, T.L., Roffman, R.A., Soloman, L.J., Winet, R.A., and Kalichman, S.C. (1997) Randomized, controlled, community-level HIV prevention and intervention for sexual risk behavior among homosexual men in US cities. *Lancet*, **350**, 1500–5.

2. Kegeles, S.M., Hays, R.B., and Coates, T.J. (1996) The Mpowerment Project: a community-level HIV prevention intervention for gay men. *Am J Public Health*, **86**(8), 1129–36.

3. Kegeles, S.M., Hays, R.B., Pollack, L.M., and Coates, T.J. (1999) Mobilizing young gay and bisexual men for HIV prevention: a two-community study. *AIDS*, **13**, 1753–62.

4. Rogers, E. (1983) *Diffusion of Innovations*. Free Press, New York.

5. Hart, G. (1998) Hope for evidence-based HIV/AIDS prevention? *AIDS*, **10**, 337–8.

6. Kelly, J.A., St Lawrence, J.S., Diaz, Y.E., Stevenson, L.Y., Hauth, A.C., Brasfield, T.L., Kalicman, S.C., Smith, J.E., and Andrew, M.E. (1991) HIV risk behaviour reduction following intervention with key opinion leaders of population: an experimental analysis. *Am J Public Health*, **81**, 168–71.

7. Kelly, J.A., St Lawrence, J.S., Stevenson, L.Y., Hauth, A.C., Kalichman, S.C., Diaz, Y.E., Brasfield, T.L., Koob, J.J., and Morgan, M.G. (1992) Community AIDS/HIV risk reduction: the effects of endorsements by popular people in three cities. *Am J Public Health*, **82**, 1483–9.

8. Kelly, J.A. (1994) HIV prevention among gay and bisexual men in small cities. In: DiClemente, R.J. and Peterson, J.L. (eds) *Preventing AIDS: Theories and Methods of Behavioural Interventions.* Plenum Press, New York, pp. 297–317.

9. Holland, J., Arnold, S., Fullerton, D., Oakley, A., and Hart, G. (1994) *Review of Effectiveness of Health Promotion Interventions for Men who have Sex with Men.* Social Science Research Unit, Institute of Education, London.

10. Flowers, P., Frankis, J.S., and Hart, G.J. (2000) Evidence and the evaluation of a community-level intervention: researching the Gay Men's Task Force initiative. In: Watson, J. and Platt, S. (eds) *Researching Health Promotion.* Routledge, London.

11. Hart, G.J., Flowers, P., Der, G.J., and Frankis, J.S. (1999) Homosexual men's HIV-related sexual risk behaviour in Scotland. *Sex Trans Infect,* **75,** 242–6.

12. Flowers, P. and Hart, G. (1999) 'Everyone on the scene is so cliquey': are gay bars an appropriate social context for a community-based peer-led intervention? In: Aggleton, P., Hart, G., and Davies, P. (eds) *Families and Communities Responding to AIDS.* Taylor and Francis, London, pp. 83–98.

13. Elford, J., Sherr, L., Bolding, G., Maguire, M., and Serle, F. (2000) Peer-led HIV prevention among gay men in London (the 4-gym project): intervention and evaluation. In: Watson, J. and Platt, S. (eds) *Researching Health Promotion.* Routledge, London.

14. Elford, J., Bolding, G., and Sherr, L. (2001) Peer education has no significant impact on HIV risk behaviours among gay men in London. *AIDS,* **15,** 1409–15.

15. Flowers, P., Hart, G.J., Williamson, L.M., Frankis, J.S., and Der, G.J. (2002) Does bar-based peer-led sexual health promotion have a community-level effect amongst gay men in Scotland? *Int J STD AIDS,* **13,** 102–8.

16. Williamson, L.M., Hart, G.J., Flowers, P., Frankis, J.S., and Der, G.J. (2001) The Gay Men's Task Force: the impact of peer education on the sexual risk behaviour of homosexual men in Glasgow. *Sex Transm Infect,* **77,** 427–32.

17. Frankis, J., Flowers, P., and Hart, G. (2002) The gay men's task force: Preliminary evaluation of service delivery. Report for Greater Glasgow Health Board 2002. MRC Medical Sociology Unit Working Paper No. 68.

18. Elford, J., Sherr, L., Bolding, G., Serle, F., and Maguire, M. (2002) Peer-led HIV prevention among gay men in London: process evaluation. *AIDS Care,* **14,** 351–60.

19. Elford, J., Hart, G., Sherr, L., Williamson, L., and Bolding, G., (2002) Peer-led HIV prevention among gay men in Britain: expanding the evidence base. *Sex Trans Infec,* **78,** 158–9.

Chapter 13

The value of systematic reviews of the effectiveness of sexual health interventions

Jonathan Shepherd and Angela Harden

Other chapters in this book consider various issues in the conduct of experimental evaluations of sexual health promotion. This chapter is concerned with bringing together the results of such experimental evaluations in the form of systematic reviews. It explores the extent to which systematic reviews are reliable and useful, and their relevance to the field of sexual health. Promoting sexual health involves what are essentially 'social' rather than clinical interventions.[1,2] Examples include educational techniques to raise awareness or develop sexual negotiation skills, and interventions to tackle structural inequalities that create and sustain unsafe sexual practices.

Three questions are addressed:

1 Why bring together the results of a number of different trials of sexual health promotion, and how might this best be done?

2 How might systematic reviews take into account the quality of the primary evaluations they include?

3 How can systematic reviews address practical issues in delivering sexual health promotion?

In relation to the first question, the focus is on methods for *synthesising* the results of several trials. Techniques such as meta-analysis and narrative synthesis are discussed and the advantages and disadvantages of each explored. The issue of heterogeneity amongst the interventions, populations and outcomes in trials is key to exploring these pros and cons. In addressing the second question, the focus is on critical appraisal of methodological quality of studies for inclusion in a systematic review. For the third question the chapter considers why process evaluation can be an important source of evidence in systematic reviews of sexual health promotion, and goes on to explore how they might be included in systematic reviews. Key issues here are the usefulness of this approach to potential users of reviews, and how the quality of process evaluation might be assessed.

The chapter makes extensive use of examples from a programme of work on evidence-based health promotion undertaken at the Evidence Informed Policy and Practice Information and Coordinating Centre (EPPI-Centre) at the Social Science Research Unit, University of London Institute of Education.

The chapter concludes with a summary of the authors' view on the value of systematic reviews of sexual health promotion and outlines some recommendations for the conduct of systematic reviews of the promotion of sexual health and health promotion in general.

Why bring together the results of several trials of sexual health promotion?

Trials of sexual health promotion aim to answer the question 'does intervention strategy x lead to positive changes in sexual health outcome y in population z?'. There are two main limitations in relying on the answer produced by a single trial: lack of sufficient precision with which the effect of an intervention can be detected, and difficulty in generalizing the results of a trial beyond the specific study participants and intervention tested.[3] In other words, the results of one trial may be spurious or due to chance and it is only by looking across trials that we can be confident in our conclusions about the effectiveness of interventions. In certain circumstances statistically combining the results of a number of averaged sized trials will boost the total sample size and potentially increase the ability to detect precisely an effect of the intervention if one exists.[4] This may be particularly useful in sexual health promotion where many evaluations do not have large enough sample sizes to show an effect.

The following examples illustrate some of the above points. Early trials of corticosteroids to prevent complications from premature birth indicated that, in general, the treatment was associated with moderate benefit, that is, fewer deaths among premature babies. It was only when all the trials were first combined in 1989, in a systematic review[5] that the extent of benefit became apparent. It is estimated that had the review been conducted earlier, the intervention would have been more widely used and thousands of premature babies would not have suffered and died unnecessarily. Similarly, in a review of smoking cessation interventions in pregnancy,[6] only 12 out of 34 trials showed a statistically significant effect on women giving up, but the pooled data from all trials showed a clear substantial benefit of intervention. In a review of the effects of commercial breastfeeding promotional materials for new mothers at hospital discharge, only two of the nine trials showed a negative impact on exclusive breastfeeding.[7] However, when the data were pooled, a significant detrimental effect was detected, namely a reduction in the period of exclusive breastfeeding. Thus, meta-analysis of health promotion interventions can be useful in detecting harm as well as benefit.

Bringing together the findings from many trials can help to establish where the effects of sexual health promotion are consistent and where they vary across different populations, settings and types of intervention.[8] This kind of information is crucial for those providing sexual health promotion services. It can also help researchers to identify gaps in knowledge about intervention effects and to plan new research.[9] Methods for bringing together the results of trials have undergone considerable development in the last few years and the 'systematic review' is considered the most rigorous technique with which to achieve this. We now explore this technique in greater detail.

What are systematic reviews?

A systematic review is 'A review of a clearly formulated question that uses systematic and explicit methods to identify, select, and critically appraise relevant research, and to collect and analyse data from the studies that are included in the review. Statistical methods (meta-analysis) may or may not be used to analyse and summarize the results of the included studies'.[10] The evidence-based health movement has led to a recent surge in systematic reviews, although the practice of combining studies is not new. There are examples of meta-analyses in the field of education and psychology from the 1970s (see Fitz-Gibbon[11] and Oakley[12] for a discussion of these). It is largely in the 1980s and 1990s that the practice has gathered momentum in the field of health, with the establishment of organizations to produce and disseminate reviews such as the Cochrane Collaboration. Systematic reviews are thus part of a broader 'movement' which aims to get high quality research evidence used in making decisions about policy and practice in health care. Such a movement is gaining rapid ground in other areas of public policy and thus social interventions are coming under the same scrutiny as clinical ones.[12,13] Sexual health promotion is an interesting example in this respect as it often involves social interventions to bring about health gain. The evidence base for sexual health promotion has recently been described as 'dispersed and unsystematic' (Department of Health (see Ref. 14, p. 17)), suggesting the need for high quality systematic reviews.

It is therefore important that all the stages of a review, as in any piece of research, are conducted in a sound and methodical way. Although the precise characteristics of reviews vary, there are usually a number of discrete stages including formulation of the review question; development of inclusion and exclusion criteria for studies; writing and publishing a protocol; searching for and retrieving reports of studies; applying inclusion and exclusion criteria to retrieved reports; extracting data and critically appraising the included studies; and combining them in some form that allows conclusions and recommendations for policy and practice. Whilst this description implies that the stages take place sequentially, in reality they often take place concurrently with data extraction and critical appraisal, for example, being conducted whilst reports are still being retrieved.

In posing the question 'what makes a review systematic?' Peersman and others[15] highlight the importance of the methods used in conducting and reporting the review 'The methods used in conducting a systematic review aim to limit both systematic errors (bias) and errors that occur by chance (random errors). These methods are explicitly reported so that others can assess the integrity of the review process, and hence, the validity of the review' (see Ref. 15, p. 136). For example, comprehensive literature searching is regarded as one of the most important factors that distinguish systematic reviews from 'traditional' reviews.[10] The aim is to locate as much relevant literature as possible to ensure that the results and conclusions of the review are based, as far as possible, on *all* of the available evidence. This will include searching for studies that may be difficult to access, for example, unpublished studies or those published in languages other than English. Without such exhaustive searching, the conclusions of the review may be biased in favour of published studies. This is particularly important as published studies tend to be more likely to conclude that interventions are effective.[16,17]

What is the best way to bring together the results of several trials in a systematic review?

There are two main ways to combine studies in a systematic review: quantitatively whereby the results of several studies are statistically pooled (e.g. meta-analysis), or qualitatively where the results are summarized and integrated using words (e.g. narrative synthesis). As we will go on to argue, there are merits and shortcomings associated with each, and they are not necessarily mutually exclusive.

In meta-analysis the results of trials are pooled to form a summary statistic or effect size, such as an 'odds ratio' (OR, the ratio of the odds of an effect happening amongst those receiving an intervention to the odds of an effect for those not receiving it), a 'relative risk' (RR, the ratio of risk for those receiving an intervention to the risk for those not receiving it), or a 'd score' (the standardized difference in means divided by the pooled standard deviation). One of the benefits of quantitative synthesis is that it does not just indicate whether an intervention works, but also the degree to which it is effective.[18] For example, 'd scores', with a value of 0.2 are considered small, 0.5 medium, and 0.8 large.[19] Whilst meta-analysis is a powerful and useful technique, misapplication can lead to results which are misleading, with potentially serious implications for policy and practice.

One of the pitfalls of this method is that interventions with a shared aim, to prevent HIV transmission, for example, may vary widely in a number of ways. To ensure that like is compared with like, the studies being combined need to be as homogeneous as possible. Methodological heterogeneity arises from differences in study design (e.g. variations in the duration of follow-up of participants), clinical heterogeneity signifies differences in participants, interventions, or outcome measures, whilst statistical heterogeneity refers to differences in reported effects between studies.

A meta-analysis of the effectiveness of condoms in preventing HIV infection illustrates how methodological heterogeneity may produce misleading results.[20] Warner and Hatcher[21] suggest that this review 'knowingly combines studies with widely different measures of condom usage' (see Ref. 21, p. 1169). Some studies measure 'method failure', the inability of the condom to prevent transmission despite being used correctly and consistently, and others assessed 'user failure', the sexual partners' inability to use it properly for every act of sexual intercourse. The conclusion of the first review was that condoms only provide 69 per cent risk reduction of HIV transmission. However, an updated review, which distinguished between user failure and method failure, concluded that consistent use of condoms results in 80 per cent reduction in HIV incidence.[22]

This raises an issue at the heart of the debate in evidence-based health promotion and systematic reviews of the effectiveness of social interventions. Can meta-analysis ever be applied appropriately to summarize the effects of these interventions? Compare a review of pharmacotherapy, for example, post exposure prophylaxis for reducing the likelihood of HIV infection in people exposed to HIV, with a review of community education approaches to preventing sexually transmitted diseases, for example, the provision of a health advice drop-in clinic, combined with outreach in community groups. The drug intervention is likely to be more 'standardized' in that the compound will be the same for everyone who takes it, regardless of where they live. In contrast, the education intervention may vary widely according to who delivers it (e.g. nurse, peer volunteer), the particular mode of delivery (e.g. one to one; small groups), the type of 'advice' given (e.g. use of condoms and other approaches to risk reduction), and the different needs of the community in question (e.g. Native American young people in the United States, south Asian teenagers living in London). Therefore, what appears to be a homogenous approach to preventing STDs is actually highly variable. Would it be appropriate to use meta-analysis to quantitatively combine all of these and conclude that education to prevent STDs is effective or ineffective to a particular degree?

The systematic review by Stephenson *et al.*[23] included studies evaluating the effectiveness of interventions to prevent STD/HIV infection. Although the studies shared a common outcome, that is, prevention of STD transmission, and were all conducted in STD clinics, they varied widely in terms of design and target population. In some cases the intervention took place in small discussion groups, in others it comprised one-to-one counseling. Interventions could last from anything between half an hour to a total of over 14 h. Some involved African American women, whilst others were targeted specifically at gay men. Given such diversity it was felt that meta-analysis of these studies was inappropriate.

An alternative would be to conduct more focused systematic reviews, which only consider one specific type of intervention, in particular 'types' of population. This is an issue of 'lumping or splitting' the scope of a review, that is, joining together or separating out its components. Thus, instead of conducting a general review of educational interventions to promote risk reduction in an unspecified population ('lumping'), a number of separate reviews ('splitting') might be carried out with specific groups (e.g. young women, injecting drug users, commercial sex workers), with particular interventions (e.g. education only, education plus skills development, risk assessment). Heterogeneity may remain even in what could be considered to be a relatively focused review. The protocol for a systematic review of interventions for preventing HIV infection in street youth (i.e. young people who are homeless, or engaged in sex work) proposes to stratify included studies according to population characteristics and type of intervention.[24] A separate meta-analysis will then be performed for each stratum. However, as the authors note, quantitative synthesis might not be appropriate in which case narrative synthesis will be undertaken.

Similar dilemmas were experienced in a review of interventions, based on social learning theory, to reduce risk behaviour for HIV.[25] An overall effect size (*d* score) was calculated for 12 trials which, as the authors acknowledge, were diverse in terms of population characteristics (e.g. pregnant women, gay and bisexual men, college students); settings (e.g. health clinics, high schools); intervention doses (20 sessions over 3 weeks; a one-off session); and evaluation methods (e.g. outcome measures). Despite the obvious heterogeneity, the studies were combined and separate analyses were performed to see whether effects varied according to the intervention doses, drop-out rates, and the interval at which outcomes were measured. Only the latter was related to effectiveness and it was suggested that the marked differences in intervention dose between studies may have had an impact on effectiveness had there been more studies in the analysis (which would have provided greater statistical power to detect an effect).

One of the useful aspects of this review was the provision of descriptive information of the included trials. The characteristics of each study were summarized in a table giving details of sample, intervention, evaluation design, and outcomes. This provides a useful context for interpreting the results, and enables the reader to judge for themselves how appropriate the chosen analysis was. This example also illustrates how meta-analytic and narrative forms of analysis might complement each other. Summary effect sizes might be useful to those who want to compare the relative effectiveness of interventions across areas, whilst narrative analysis will provide essential context, and provide specific information for those engaged in planning and providing work with particular populations.

If meta-analysis is deemed inappropriate, a narrative form of synthesis may be undertaken. Key study characteristics may be presented in tabular form (e.g. mode of intervention delivery, socio-demographic profile of participants) alongside the study findings about the effect of the intervention. A narrative would then be used to summarize findings, highlighting similarities and differences in study characteristics. For example, a review might summarize the results of each intervention and note that whilst a number of studies demonstrated positive changes in knowledge and attitudes about sexual risk reduction, fewer demonstrated changes in sexual negotiation skills. The review may then go on to describe in detail the circumstances under which interventions were found to have positive effects, negative effects, or no effects. When relying solely on narrative synthesis, reviews must be careful to avoid simple 'vote counting' of the number of significant positive or negative findings in order to draw overall conclusions about the effects of an intervention. A number of drawbacks of this technique have been identified.[26] In particular, vote-counting does not take into account sample size or the size of an effect. When sample sizes are large, there is a higher probability of detecting a significant effect even if the actual effect is very small. Conversely, when sample sizes are small, it is much more difficult to detect a significant effect even if one exists. Thus a review which concludes that sexual health promotion does not work because the majority of trials do not show statistically significant effects may be misleading if these trials are small studies of low power. A meta-analysis of these studies, if appropriate, may well detect a significant positive effect. With any method of synthesis, its quality ultimately depends on the methodological quality of the studies being synthesized. As Stephenson[27] notes in relation to statistical meta-analysis, although it might be a powerful technique, it cannot address the problems of bias present in the original studies. We deal with issues of methodological quality in systematic reviews next.

How do we ensure systematic reviews take into account the quality of studies?

To be confident about the findings of a systematic review, the design and conduct of the review must be sound. In particular, the quality of individual studies must be assessed to ensure the recommendations and conclusions are based on sound evidence. Empirical studies have shown that non-randomized trials can lead to significantly different conclusions compared with randomized controlled trials (RCTs). In general, non-randomized trials tend to overestimate the effectiveness of interventions in comparison to RCTs and thereby risk labelling an ineffective or harmful intervention as effective.[28] Guyatt *et al.*[29] compared the results of 13 RCTs with 17 non-randomized trials of the effectiveness of interventions to prevent pregnancy amongst young people. They found that the non-randomized trials consistently overestimated the effect of the interventions compared to RCTs. The authors argued that this finding could not be explained by factors such as the quality of the interventions (it seemed unlikely that the randomized trials evaluated poorer interventions than the non-randomized trials), secular changes in pregnancy rates, or differences in duration of follow-up. The authors concluded that the most likely explanation for the result was that the young people who were non-randomly assigned to an intervention group in the non-randomized trials were already predisposed to better outcomes regardless of the intervention, that is, that those most likely to use birth control were more willing to participate in the intervention and vice versa. Studies such as this provide powerful evidence against relying on non-randomized studies for evaluation of effectiveness.

It is therefore important to take a critical view of the evidence in systematic reviews because biases in the primary studies may bias the findings of the review. Methodological quality can be considered at various key stages in the review process, including searching for studies, setting the inclusion criteria, extracting data from included studies, and combining the results of the studies. From the outset it may be decided that only certain types of studies, or studies with specified methodological attributes, may be included in a review. The Cochrane HIV/AIDS Collaborative Review Group, for example, which conducts reviews on prevention and treatment, states that it includes 'rigorous studies of different designs' including controlled trials, both randomized and non-randomized, as well as interrupted time series studies.[30]

Critical appraisal is still necessary if the review protocol specifies that only 'rigorous' evidence, that is, RCTs should be included. However, this approach is not always adopted. In a review of around 400 reviews (systematic and non-systematic) of the effectiveness of health promotion, two-thirds of reviews weighted the findings according to strengths and weaknesses of study design, but only a third explicitly indicated the criteria that had been used.[31] It is important to describe the methods used to assess quality of studies to enable the reader to judge whether this was done systematically. If the assessment is not systematic, certain studies may be singled out for criticism, thereby biasing the findings of the review.

Opinion varies considerably on what constitutes sound evidence for the effectiveness of sexual health promotion. This reflects wider debates about evidence in the field of health promotion and social interventions.[2,32–35] Whilst some take RCTs to be the 'gold standard', others consider a range of different evaluation designs to be appropriate. Consequently, there is little consensus on what criteria should be employed to judge evaluations in systematic reviews.

For example, the review of interventions to prevent HIV/AIDS delivered in the workplace by Wilson et al.[36] employed a hierarchy of evidence rating studies on a five-point scale, with RCTs scoring the highest, and anecdotal evidence or expert opinion the lowest. Other methodological attributes take into account whether the sample was representative, the response and drop out rates, the reliability and validity of the instruments used to measure outcomes, and whether or not the data analysis was appropriate.

Stephenson and others[23] in their methodological review of RCTs of interventions to prevent STD/HIV considered a number of dimensions of quality including the size of the trial, method of randomization, how outcomes were defined and measured (e.g. sensitivity of diagnostic tests) and completeness of follow-up. The review of educational interventions for contraceptive use for women after childbirth by Hiller and Griffith[30] likewise prioritised RCTs (using random or quasi-random allocation methods) and also assessed whether the method of randomization was appropriate, how it was concealed from participants, and whether blinding was achieved.

In contrast a review by Stanton et al.[37] employed fewer criteria: whether or not study participants had been randomly assigned to groups, and whether or not pre- and post-intervention data on outcomes had been collected. These criteria do not, however, take into account other aspects of methodological quality, such as whether or not the study groups were balanced in terms of socio-demographic or outcome measures at the start of the trial, or the level of drop out. In other words, there is little here to distinguish between a 'good' RCT and a 'bad' one.

Many sexual health interventions have been poorly evaluated. Several reviews in this area[1,2,38,39] have identified a relatively small number of methodologically sound studies from the literature. For example, in a review of interventions to prevent HIV/AIDS by Oakley et al.[2] only around a quarter of all studies assessed were judged to be methodologically sound (18 out of 68). In a review of the effectiveness of sexual health promotion interventions for young people by Peersman et al.[38] the difference was even larger with just under a fifth of studies being judged methodologically sound (21 of 110, 19%).

How can systematic reviews address practical issues in delivering sexual health promotion?

The importance of evaluating process alongside outcome is being increasingly highlighted in the health promotion evaluation literature (e.g. Davies and MacDonald[40], Oakley[41], Speller et al.,[35] see also Bonell and Oakley, and Wight and Obasi, this volume). Some recent trials in the United Kingdom have adopted this approach (Elford et al.,[42] Imrie et al.,[43] Strange et al.,[44] Wight and Abraham.[45]) In contrast with outcome evaluation, process evaluation is not designed to answer questions about effectiveness, but rather to describe the way and the context in which interventions are delivered. Process evaluation is frequently used to explain why the intervention was successful or unsuccessful and whether the intervention was implemented as intended. It often, though not exclusively, uses qualitative methods of data collection and analysis such as in-depth interviews or observation.

There is growing interest in developing methods for including process evaluations and other qualitative studies in systematic reviews (e.g. Dixon-Woods and Fitzpatrick,[46] Murphy et al.[47]). Indeed, Speller et al.[35] argue that because process evaluation can shed light on the quality of the *intervention*, it should be given more attention in health promotion systematic reviews. For example, in a trial testing a particular sex education curriculum implemented across a number of different schools, a process evaluation might look for differences in the skills of those providing the intervention. Users of systematic reviews such as health promotion practitioners have emphasized that presentation of process data alongside outcome data is a critical factor in making systematic reviews useful.[31,48] This may help users to determine how to implement an effective intervention, whether it is transferable to their particular context, whether it is likely to be acceptable and accessible to their population group, and on whose terms intervention success has been determined. Indeed, it could be argued that unless an intervention and its implementation is adequately described and monitored, it may be of limited use to know whether or not it is effective. This kind of analysis may help unpack the various factors that may influence the impact of an intervention, and help determine the homogeneity or heterogeneity of interventions in a systematic review.

So, how might process evaluation be included in systematic reviews of effectiveness? There are currently very few examples of reviews which set out to integrate the findings of outcome evaluations with those from process evaluations. This section therefore draws on the insights gained from a review of peer-delivered health promotion (including sexual health promotion) for young people, reported in Harden et al.[49] This review aimed to examine the appropriateness, as well as the effectiveness, of this type of intervention and to synthesize systematically the findings from both process and outcome evaluations. The methods used in process evaluation are different from outcome evaluation and they address different data, such as the themes that emerge from analysis of interview transcripts or analysis of field and observation notes describing the context or delivery of an intervention. The review therefore adapted the procedures for systematic reviews of effectiveness research, being careful to maintain the key principles of systematic review methodology outlined in the previous sections.

Searching identified a total of 49 outcome evaluations which met the inclusion criteria for the review of which only 12 were of sufficient methodological quality to generate potentially reliable conclusions about effectiveness. Of these only three carried out integral process evaluations. This suggests a traditional distinction between conducting either process or outcome evaluations, but rarely both. Other work[8] has shown that only 15 per cent (222/1497) of evaluative reports collected for potential inclusion in various systematic reviews of effectiveness in health promotion (including sexual health promotion) collected both outcome and process data.

The searches for the review of peer-delivered interventions also identified 15 evaluations of process only which met the review's inclusion criteria. The findings were synthesized with the 12 methodologically sound outcome evaluations to draw conclusions about the effectiveness and appropriateness of this peer-led health promotion. A narrative synthesis of the outcome evaluations showed uncertainty about the effectiveness of the method. It was not possible to specify an effective model of peer education. No consistent relationships were found between effectiveness and the different characteristics of interventions such as age of peer leaders, methods used to recruit them or the particular 'model' of peer education used (e.g. simply using peer leaders to deliver an intervention designed by professionals or engaging peer leaders as partners in developing as well as delivering the intervention). This unclear picture was compounded by the heterogeneity of interventions and the young people studied, and the lack of detail on the intervention presented in the outcome evaluations.

However, the synthesis of the findings from the process evaluations helped to provide insight into issues affecting the implementation of peer-delivered health promotion and its acceptability to young people. In particular, the organizational context in which interventions were implemented seemed to have a significant impact on the functioning of peer-delivered health promotion. A common problem identified was the conflict between peer education being regarded as a non-traditional educational strategy, but being implemented in traditional school settings. Peer leaders might then be seen as 'teachers' while teachers might undermine peer leaders' control over the content and organization of their sessions. These insights were used to make recommendations for the further development and evaluation of potentially effective interventions. One strength of including process evaluations in this systematic review therefore lay in helping to set a future research agenda against a meagre background of good evaluations. For another example of how to integrate process data with outcome data in a systematic review, see Oliver and Peersman.[50]

One of the challenges faced in this review was how to assess the methodological quality of the process evaluations. Since there is little consensus about how to assess the validity and reliability of qualitative methods, criteria proposed by four research groups[12] were examined and seven criteria were applied independently by two reviewers. The seven criteria were: explicit and clear description of theoretical framework and/or literature review; aims; context; sample used and sample methods; data collection and analysis methods; attempts to establish reliability and/or validity of data analysis; inclusion of sufficient data for mediation between data and interpretation. Applying these criteria was not easy; there was seldom enough detail to allow reviewers to judge whether the findings of the process evaluations were an artifact of the particular methods or samples used. Only two process evaluations met all seven quality criteria. More empirical work is required to test these and other criteria for their ability to identify those studies which are capable of producing the most reliable findings about process.

Conclusions

This chapter has explored a number of key issues that relate to the usefulness of systematic reviews, including the appropriateness of different forms of synthesis, ensuring conclusions are supported by sound evidence, and broadening the types of evidence included in reviews. However, there are important limitations associated with representing the effectiveness of diverse initiatives by a single numerical measure. Misleading conclusions may be reached if such limitations are not taken into account. Narrative forms of syntheses can be supplementary to techniques such as meta-analysis, but they are particularly valuable in their own right. However, this form of synthesis has its own drawbacks. Ideally a combination of the two should be used to enhance the appeal of reviews to different users.

The incorporation of data from process evaluation has the potential to boost a review's explanatory power, and can help to determine whether interventions are sufficiently homogenous to warrant meta-analysis. At present, there are very few rigorous evaluations that have collected process and outcome data, although there are signs that this is changing.

Critical appraisal of primary evaluation methodology is absolutely vital to ensure systematic reviews do not inherit the biases of the studies they include. Although randomized controlled trials have been carried out in the field of sexual health promotion, many evaluations have suffered from methodological shortcomings, reflecting some of the problems inherent in the evaluation of social interventions. The challenge for future research is to establish ways of conducting more stringent evaluation.

Acknowledgements

We would like to thank Greet Peersman and Sandy Oliver for commenting on drafts of this chapter, and colleagues at the EPPI-Centre for thoughtful discussion and debate. Thanks also to Sandy Oliver for highlighting reviews that illustrate discrepancies between individual trials and pooled trials. The Department of Health (DoH), England, funds a specific programme of work on evidence-based health promotion at the EPPI-Centre. The views expressed in this publication are those of the authors and not necessarily those of the DoH.

References

1. Oakley, A. and Fullerton, D. (1996) The lamp-post of research: support or illumination? The case for and against randomized controlled trials. In: Oakley, A. and Roberts, H. (eds) *Evaluating Social Interventions*. Barnados, Ilford, Essex.

2. Oakley, A., Fullerton, D., Holland, J., Arnold, S., France-Dawson, M., Kelley, P., and McGrellis, S. (1995) Sexual health education interventions for young people: a methodological review. *Br Med J*, **310**, 158–62.

3. Thompson, S.G. and Pocock, S.J. (1991) Can meta-analyses be trusted? *Lancet*, **338**(8775), 1127–30.

4. Dickersin, K. and Berlin, J. (1992) Meta-analysis: state of the science. *Epidemiol Rev*, **14**, 154–76.

5. Crowley, P. (1989) Promoting pulmonary maternity. In: Chalmers, I., Enkin, M., and Keirse M.J.N.C. (eds) *Effective Care in Pregnancy and Childbirth*. Oxford University Press, Oxford. pp. 746–64.

6. Lumley, J., Oliver, S., and Waters, E. (2002) Interventions for promoting smoking cessation during pregnancy (Cochrane Review). Issue 1, Oxford: Update Software.

7. Donnelly, A., Snowden, H.M., Renfrew, M.J., and Woolridge, M.W. (2002) Commercial hospital discharge packs for breastfeeding women (Cochrane Review). Issue 1 Oxford: Update Software.

8. Peersman, G. and Oakley, A. (2001) Learning from research. In: Oliver, S. and Peersman, G. (eds) *Using Research for Effective Health Promotion*. Open University Press, Buckingham.

9. Petticrew, M. (2001) Systematic reviews from astronomy to zoology: myths and misconceptions. *Br Med J* **322**, 98–101.

10. Clarke, M. and Oxman, A.D. (2001) *Cochrane Reviewers Handbook 4.1* (updated March 2001), In: *The Cochrane Library*, Issue 2, Oxford.

11. Fitz-Gibbon, C. (1985) The implications of meta-analysis for educational research. *Br Educ Res J*, **11**, 45–9.

12. Oakley, A. (2000) *Experiments in Knowing: Gender & Method in the Social Sciences*. Polity, Cambridge.

13. Davies, H., Nutley, S., and Smith, P. (2000) *What Works? Evidence-based Policy and Practice in Public Services*. The Policy Press, Bristol.

14. Department of Health. *The National Strategy for Sexual Health and HIV*. HMSO, London.

15. Peersman, G., Oliver, S., and Oakley, A. (2001) Systematic reviews of effectiveness. In: Oliver, S. and Peersman, G. *Using Research for Effective Health Promotion*. Open University Press, Buckingham.

16. Dickersin, K., Chan, S., Chalmers, T., Sacks Jr, H. (1987) Publication bias and clinical trials. *Control Clin Trials*, (8), 343–53.

17. Dickersin, K. (1997) How important is publication bias? *AIDS Educ Prev*, **9**(Suppl. A): 15–21.

18. Durlack, J. and Lipsey, M. (1991) A practitioner's guide to meta-analysis. *Am J Community Psychol*, **19**(3), 291–332.

19. Cohen, J. (1977) *Statistical Power Analysis for the Behavioural Sciences*. Academic Press, New York.

20. Weller, S. (1993) A meta-analysis of condom effectiveness in reducing sexually transmitted diseases. *Soc Sci Med*, **36**(12), 1635–44.

21. Warner, D. and Hatcher, R. (1994) A meta-analysis of condom effectiveness in reducing sexually transmitted diseases (Letter). *Soc Sci Med*, **38**(8), 1169–70.

22. Weller, S. and Davis, S. (2001) Condom effectiveness in reducing heterosexual HIV transmission (Cochrane Review). In: *The Cochrane Library*, Issue 3, Oxford.

23. Stephenson, J.M., Imrie, J., and Sutton, S.R. (2000) Rigorous trials of sexual behaviour interventions in STD/HIV prevention: what can we learn from them? *AIDS*, **14**(suppl. 3): S115–S124.

24. Grossman, D.W., Arbess, G., Cavacuiti, C., and Urbshott, G.B. (2001) Interventions for preventing HIV infection in street youth (Protocol for a Cochrane Review). In: *The Cochrane Library*, Issue 3, Oxford.

25. Kalichman, S.C., Carey, M.P., and Johnson, B.T. (2001) Prevention of sexually transmitted HIV infection: a meta-analytic review of the behavioural outcomes literature. *Soc Behav Med*, **18**(1), 6–15.

26. Bushman, B. (1994) Vote-counting procedures in meta-analysis. In Copper, H. and Hedges, L. (eds) *The Handbook of Research Synthesis*. Russell Sage Foundation, New York.

27. Stephenson, J. (1998) Systematic review of steroid contraceptives and risk of HIV transmission: when to resist meta-analysis. *AIDS*, **12**, 545–53.

28. Kleijnen, J., Gotzsche, P., Kunz, R.A., Oxman, A., and Chalmers, I. (1997) So what's so special about randomization? In Maynard, A. and Chalmers, I. (eds) *Non-random Reflections on Health Services Research*. BMJ Publishing Group, London.

29. Guyatt, G.H., DiCenso, A., Farewell, V., Willan, A., and Griffith, L. (2000) Randomized trials versus observational studies in adolescent pregnancy prevention. *J Clin Epidemiol*, **53**, 167–74.

30. Hiller, J.E. and Griffith, E. (2001) Education for contraceptive use by women after childbirth (Cochrane Review). In: *The Cochrane Library*, Issue 3, Oxford.

31. Peersman, G., Harden, A., Oliver, S., and Oakley, A. (1999) *Effectiveness of Reviews in Health Promotion*. EPI-Centre, London.

32. Macintyre, S. and Petticrew, M. (2000) Good intentions and wisdom are not enough. *J Epidemiol Community Health*, **54**(11), 802–3.

33. Nutbeam, D. and Oakley, A. (1999) Case for using randomised controlled trials is misleading. *Br Med J*, **318**, 944–5.

34. Nutbeam, D. (2001) Assessing the effectiveness of public health interventions. *Evidence into practice: Challenges and Opportunities for UK Public Health*—Conference. Oral presentation at Health Development Agency & King's Fund, London, 3 April 2001.

35. Speller, V., Learmonth, A., and Harrison, D. (1997) The search for evidence of effective health promotion. *Br Med J*, **315**, 361–3.

36. Wilson, M.G., Jorgensen, C., and Cole, G. (1996) The health effects of worksite HIV/AIDS interventions: a review of the research literature. *Am J Health Promot*, **11**(2), 150–7.

37. Stanton, B., Kim, N., and Galbraith, J. (1996) Design issues addressed in published evaluations of adolescent HIV risk reduction interventions: a review. *J Adolesc Health*, **18**, 387–96.

38. Peersman, G., Oakley, A., Oliver, S., and Thomas, J. (1996) Review of effectiveness of sexual health promotion interventions for young people. EPI-Centre, London.

39. Shepherd, J., Peersman, G., Weston, R., and Napuli, I. (2000) Cervical cancer and sexual lifestyle: a systematic review of health education interventions targeted at women. *Health Educ Res*, **15**(6), 681–94.

40. Davies, J.K. and MacDonald, G. (1998) Beyond uncertainty: leading health promotion into the twenty first century. In: MacDonald, J. and Davies, G. (eds) *Quality, Evidence and Effectiveness in Health Promotion*. Routledge, London.

41. Oakley, A. (2001) Evaluating health promotion. In: Oliver, S. and Peersman, G. (eds) *Using research for effective health promotion*. Open University Press, Buckingham.

42. Elford, J., Bolding, G., and Sherr, L. (2001) Peer education has no significant impact on HIV risk behaviours among gay men in London. *AIDS*, **15**(4), 535–8.

43. Imrie, J., Stephenson, J.M., Cowan, F.M., Wanigaratne, S., Billington, A.J.P., Copas, A.J., French, L., French, P.D., and Johnson, A.M. for the Behavioural Intervention in Gay Men Project Study Group. (2001) A cognitive behavioural intervention to reduce sexually transmitted infections among gay men: randomized trial. *Br Med J*, **322**, 1451–6.

44. **Strange, V., Forrest, S., and Oakley, A.** (2001) A listening trial: 'qualitative' methods within experimental research. In: Oliver, S. and Peersman, G. (eds) *Using Research for Effective Health Promotion.* Open University Press, Buckingham.

45. **Wight, D. and Abraham, C.** (2000) From psychosocial theory to sustainable classroom practice: developing a research based teacher delivered sex education programme. *Health Educ Res Theory Pract,* **15**, 25–38.

46. **Dixon-Woods, M. and Fitzpatrick, R.** (2001) Qualitative research in systematic reviews. *Br Med J,* **323**, 765–6.

47. **Murphy, E., Dingwall, R., Greatbach, D., Parker, S., and Watson, P.** (1998) *Qualitative Research Methods in Health Technology Assessment: A Review of the Literature.* National Co-ordinating Centre for Health Technology Assessment, Southampton.

48. **Oliver, S.** (2001) Making research more useful: integrating different perspectives and different study designs. In: Oliver, S. and Peersman, G. (eds) *Using Research for Effective Health Promotion.* Open University Press, Buckingham.

49. **Harden, A., Oakley, A., and Oliver, S.** (2001) Peer-delivered health promotion for young people: systematic review of different study designs. *Health Educ J,* **60**, 339–53.

50. **Oliver, S. and Peersman, G.** (2001) *Using Research for Effective Health Promotion.* Open University Press, Buckingham.

Chapter 14

Challenges for future sexual health intervention trials

Judith Stephenson

The early chapters of this book present strong arguments in favour of randomized controlled trials of sexual health interventions, and an equally vigorous rebuttal of their use in this field. Since both the trials and the debate about their value are likely to continue for the foreseeable future, the purpose of this book has been to dissect the debate and to consider how we might increase the usefulness of future trials.

As the opening sentence of Chapter 11 states, these trials have no end in themselves. They are intended as a means of improving the sexual health of people in the future. We should therefore ask how successful such trials have been in this regard. In one area of HIV prevention, conventional clinical trials have brought impressive benefits. Since the first large trial of zidovudine to reduce mother-to-child HIV transmission was published in 1994,[1] several trials have shown that other antiretroviral regimens are effective in different settings, and where these interventions are available, mother-to-child transmission of HIV has been reduced.[2] By contrast, it is unfortunately true that relatively few sexual behaviour interventions have been rigorously evaluated and shown to be effective in improving sexual health outcomes.[3] Both sides of the randomized controlled trials (RCT) debate can agree with this observation, but they respond to it quite differently. Proponents of RCTs conclude that we need more well-designed trials, while opponents interpret this as evidence that we should stop doing trials altogether rather than do more. Which is right? Are we really barking up the wrong tree, or have the trials not yet had a fair trial?

The arguments put forward by Kippax (Chapter 2) for not doing trials in this field can also be interpreted as explanations for the limited success of such trials to date. By comparison with, say, trials of antihypertensive drugs to prevent stroke, behavioural intervention trials to prevent HIV face formidable challenges. The occurrence of HIV infection over time (or incidence) is much more dynamic than stroke. Due to the pattern of spread of communicable disease epidemics, HIV incidence can increase and decrease rapidly in the absence of any intervention.[4] This makes the timing of trials in relation to the stage of the epidemic more critical and underlines the importance of evaluating interventions against control groups. Behavioural intervention trials have to work with the sexual partners and networks through which sexually communicable infections spread, unlike the non-communicable conditions of hypertension and stroke (see Chapters 3 and 7). They also have to deal with more complex causal pathways between intervention and outcome, as discussed in Chapters 8 and 9.

Clearly, behavioural interventions do not change behaviour in the way that drugs change blood pressure. People can be oblivious to the effects of their blood pressure treatment. But behavioural interventions provide the means, such as greater knowledge, choice or skill, that allow people to change their own behaviour. Another rather obvious difference between hypertension and sex has important implications for the evaluation of interventions: it is difficult to reduce high blood pressure much without medical intervention, which is not the case for sexual risk behaviour. An antihypertensive drug trial can be designed with the expectation that blood pressure levels in the control group will remain reasonably stable. In a behavioural intervention trial, people in the control group have the potential to reduce their sexual risk behaviour as much as the intervention group. And ethically they should be encouraged to do so. This is more likely to happen in long term trials where the effects of the HIV epidemic are deeply felt. In the community randomized HIV prevention trial in rural Uganda, described in Chapter 7, there was an increase in condom use and reduction in casual partners in the control group as well as in the intervention groups.[5] Similar experience has been reported in other fields of health promotion. For example, large, well-conducted community trials of cardiovascular risk reduction have reported apparently unimpressive results.[6] Susser[6] and Kippax (Chapter 2) both make the point that sustained change in risk behaviour, whether cardiovascular or sexual, takes time and is most likely to occur when supported by political will and structural change. Kippax interprets this as evidence that sexual health promotion is inherently unsuited to experimental evaluation; Susser, by contrast, argues that 'we should not abandon community trials, but should gather the knowledge necessary to refine them.' He concludes that future trials will need to draw on a deeper understanding of methods for bringing about social change. Although Kippax argues against experimental evaluation in this field, she writes, in a similar vein, about interventions needing to be 'aimed at the social glue, the stuff that binds people and groups together.'

A few large, well-designed and carefully conducted trials of sexual behaviour interventions have shown no significant effect on behavioural outcomes.[7] This includes RCTs of school-based sex education, and yet we do not relinquish the view that sex education is important. Nor should we. By analogy, it is not uncommon for more conventional, well-designed clinical trials to show that a new treatment does not work, as has happened in Alzheimer's disease. This does not mean that drug treatment of that condition is rejected. However, if we wish to improve the value of future sexual health intervention trials, then we have to face some difficult questions and challenges. Are we testing interventions that are simply inadequate? Are we failing to measure their effects accurately? Are we doing the trials at the wrong time? The HIV prevention trial in rural Uganda may be an example of the right trial done at the wrong time.

The concept of an adequate intervention needs consideration. Some of the unimpressive results of 'good' trials may reflect evaluation of interventions that are inadequate in terms of theoretical basis, formative research, intensity or duration (see Chapters 4, 5 and 12). It is probably unreasonable to expect single component interventions, such as education alone, to achieve behaviour change. Should we then focus on trialling complex (or joined up) interventions that combine clinical, health promotion and social policy interventions? Against this view, it is often argued that trials of complex interventions fail to identify the active ingredient, the component that produces most of the desired effect. But if we believe, as argued above, that sustained behaviour change at population level requires a multifaceted approach, attempts to identify an active ingredient may be fruitless. Even in pharmacological medicine, there are few magic bullets, and some antihypertensive drugs have achieved impressive reductions in mortality and morbidity that cannot be explained by their effect on blood pressure alone.[8] However, there is a more practical constraint to trialling complex interventions: the more extensive they become, the harder it is to ensure comparison groups. Interventions that, for example, encompass mass media campaigns and legislative change would be hard to evaluate against appropriate control groups. We therefore need to think carefully about what constitutes an adequate and trialable intervention.

People clearly can and do change their sexual behaviour and reduce their risk of STI regardless of health promotion interventions. Kippax argues that we should try to identify the reasons for behaviour change by observation and explore the 'social glue' that produces changes in beliefs, values and practices. Better understanding of the social glue would undoubtedly be useful, especially if that understanding could be channelled into developing better interventions. But it is hard to see how understanding the glue could replace the need for trials. As long as we wish to intervene to improve sexual health, and not just observe the factors that determine or undermine sexual health, we should make the process and outcome of our intervention as interpretable as possible, and that includes doing randomized trials. RCTs of sexual behaviour interventions may face formidable challenges, but they are undoubtedly better than other study designs at attributing change in outcome to an applied intervention.

Clinical trial methodology has developed greatly since the early trials of the 1960s, and has had much longer to evolve than sexual behaviour interventions which only became a major public health issue when the AIDS pandemic emerged in the 1980s. An optimistic view of the future for complex intervention trials is given by Haynes who argues that it is still early days for such trials.[9] According to his view, we are simply going through an evolutionary phase in testing interventions. Having 'learned to walk' with conventional trials of treatment efficacy, we are now 'learning to run—with community trials that tackle difficult challenges in research design and implementation that can undermine the feasibility of a study or prejudice the interpretation of its findings.'

One of the major challenges for future behavioural intervention trials is to speed the evolution of the interventions themselves. The development of promising interventions has less to do with RCTs than with good exploratory research. Can the glue, to which Kippax refers, be hardened into cement with which to build the right intervention? Should we try harder to adopt the MRC framework (described in Chapter 5) for the development and evaluation of complex interventions? It seems a sensible and logical approach, but it requires substantial amounts of time and money. Stakeholders may need to be more convinced that this approach will pay off in the long term.

This chapter started with a reminder that trials have no end in themselves. To be useful, they must be relevant to other, future populations. Kippax questions the usefulness of health promotion trials on the basis that what works now may not work in a few years time. She argues that health promotion trials are at greater risk of becoming out of date than drug trials because the effectiveness of a drug is the same whether it is taken this year or some other year. In fact, drug trials do become out of date, and this is particularly true in the HIV field. It does not, however, mean that earlier trials do not provide useful information, nor does it lead to a rejection of trial methodology. For example, an early placebo-controlled trial of the anti-HIV drug zidovudine is redundant now, in the sense that single drug therapy has been superseded by combined drug therapy, but it was very useful in showing that trials should not rely solely on surrogate markers like CD4 (white blood) cells because such markers can suggest benefit that is not borne out by better health outcomes.[10] We reached a similar conclusion following review of HIV/STI prevention trials that tended to show benefit in terms of reported behaviours without a reduction in STI.[3]

The requirement to make research findings relevant to future populations is a general one that applies to trials and other study designs. It is not in itself an argument for favouring one type of research method over another. To help meet this requirement, sexual behaviour trials should include assessment of contextual factors that are likely to limit or enhance the relevance of the trial now and in the future (see Chapters 10 and 11). Maximizing the relevance or utility of large HIV prevention trials is important because, as this book makes clear, such trials are very demanding and undertaken relatively infrequently. This increases the onus to maximize the potential benefit from each one. Such a utilitarian approach requires proper involvement of relevant stakeholders at the beginning, to ensure that the results of the trial will be useful to as many people and agencies as possible.

In conclusion, it is hard to see how policy-makers, service providers and educators would be better served by *not* doing trials. But it is clear that many health promotion trials to date, including those in HIV/STI prevention, have been of poor quality.[11-14] Too many reviews have concluded that it is not possible to draw firm conclusions about which interventions work and which do not, because of methodological flaws in the conception, design, conduct, and analysis of the available studies. The ultimate challenge is to ensure that systematic reviews of sexual behaviour intervention trials conducted over the next decade do not conclude that the quality of trials in this area remains poor, or that few interventions have been rigorously evaluated and shown to be effective in improving sexual health.

References

1. Connor, E.M., Sperling, R.S., Gelber, R., Kiselev, P., Scott, G., O'Sullivan, M.J., *et al.* (1994) Reduction of maternal-infant transmission of human immunodeficiency virus type 1 with zidovudine treatment. *N Engl J Med*, **331**, 1173–80.

2. Lindegren, M.L., Byers, R.H., Thomas, P., Davis, S.F., Caldwell, B., Rogers, R., *et al.* (1994) Trends in perinatal transmission of HIV/AIDS in the United States. *JAMA*, **282**, 531–8.

3. Stephenson, J.M., Imrie, J., and Sutton, S.R. (2000) Rigorous trials of sexual behaviour interventions in STD/HIV prevention: what can we learn from them? *AIDS*, **14**, S115–S124.

4. Anderson, R.M. and Garnett, G.P. (2002) Mathematical models of the transmission and control of sexually transmitted diseases. *AIDS*, **27**, 636–43.

5. Kamali, A., Quigley, M., Nakiyingi, J., *et al.* (2002) A community randomised trial of sexual behaviour and syndromic STI management interventions or HIV-1 transmission in rural Uganda. *Lancet* (in press).

6. Susser, M. (ed.) (1995) The tribulations of trials—intervention in communities. *Am J Public Health*, **85**, 156–9.

7. Guyatt, G.H., DiCenso, A., Farewell, V., Willan, A., and Griffith, L. (2000) Randomised trials versus observational studies in adolescent pregnancy prevention. *J Clin Epidemiol*, **53**, 167–74.

8. Sleight, P., Yusuf, S., Pogue, J., Tsuyuki, R., Diaz, R., Probstfield, J., *et al.* (2001) Blood-pressure reduction and cardiovascular risk in HOPE study. *Lancet*, **358**, 2130–1.

9. Haynes, B. (2000) Can it work? Does it work? Is it worth it? The testing of health care interventions is evolving. *Br Med J*, **319**, 652–3.

10. Concorde Coordinating Committee. (1994) Concorde: MRC/ANRS randomised double-blind controlled trial of immediate and deferred zidovudine in symptom-free HIV infection. *Lancet*, **343**, 871–81.

11. Oakley, A., Fullerton, D., Holland, J., Arnold, S., France-Dawson, M., Kelley, P., *et al.*, (1995) Sexual health education interventions for young people: a methodological review. *Br Med J*, **310**, 158–62.

12. Oakley, A., Fullerton, D., and Holland, J. (1995) Behavioural interventions for HIV/AIDS prevention. *AIDS*, **9**, 479–86.

13. Mellanby, A., Rees, J.B., and Tripp, J.H. (2000) Peer-led and adult-led school health education: a critical review of available comparative research. *Health Educ Res*, **15**, 533–45.

14. Harden, A., Oakley, A., and Oliver, S. (2001) Peer-delivered health promotion for young people: a systematic review of different study designs. *Health Educ J*, **60**, 339–53.

Glossary

cluster A geographically-delineated grouping of individuals (e.g. a school or a town). Cluster-controlled trials involve the allocation of such groupings, rather than of individuals, to intervention and control groups.

control group A group of trial participants allocated to experience some condition other than the intervention being evaluated (usually no intervention or the current routine intervention) for the purposes of comparison with the intervention in question. Also known as the comparison group.

controlled trial A research study in which participants are allocated to intervention (or 'experimental') and control (or 'comparison') groups, enabling comparison of the processes and outcomes experienced within each. Allocation may occur using random or non-random methods.

effectiveness An intervention achieving its key aims in terms of having demonstrable and significant beneficial effects on a specific population when deployed under routine conditions.

experimental evaluation An approach to evaluation in which participants are randomly allocated to intervention (or 'experimental') and control (or 'comparison') groups, enabling comparison of the processes and outcomes experienced within each. This approach is synonymous with use of a randomized controlled trial.

formative Evaluation, or other research, that is conducted in order to maximize the appropriateness, acceptability and consistency of an intervention, often prior to an evaluation of the intervention's effectiveness.

health promotion Activities that aim to enable populations to achieve greater control and improve their health via addressing the factors that determine their health.

intention-to-treat analysis Analysis of a controlled trial wherein participants are compared according to whether they were allocated to the intervention or control group, regardless of subsequent experience.

interpretivism The proposition that research on social phenomena (e.g. sexual risk-taking) should explore how the people concerned (e.g. those at risk) themselves interpret these phenomena, rather than trying to examine the phenomena externally and objectively.

intervention group A group of participants allocated to experience the intervention under evaluation. Also known as the experimental group.

matching A non-random method used to ensure the comparability, with regard to those characteristics regarded as most predictive of key outcomes, of intervention and control groups within a quasi-experimental evaluation.

meta-analysis A statistical method by which the quantitative findings of a number of studies, deemed to be very similar in focus and methods, are pooled to enable the production of quantitative summary.

narrative review A method by which the quantitative and/or qualitative findings of a number studies, deemed to be broadly similar in focus and methods, are collated and discussed so as to provide a qualitative summary.

on-treatment analysis Analysis of a controlled trial wherein participants are compared according to which intervention, if any, they experienced, regardless of initial allocation.

outcome measure A pre-specified indicator of the effect of an intervention upon participants, intended to enable an assessment of whether that intervention is effective in achieving key aims.

positivism The proposition that research, regardless of whether it investigates natural or social phenomena, should aim to develop objective accounts, describe general patterns, elucidate causal relationships and construct laws enabling prediction of future events.

process The means by which an intervention is delivered and/or received.

qualitative data Data that provide a description of a phenomenon using non-numeric information.

quantitative data Data that provide a description of a phenomenon using numeric information.

quasi-experimental evaluation An approach to evaluation in which intervention and control groups are employed, but the composition of these is not determined randomly.

randomization The allocation of participants to intervention or control group using methods that ensure that chance, rather than any attribute of the participants or investigators, determines allocation.

randomized controlled trial An experimental evaluation design in which participants are randomly allocated to intervention (or 'experimental') and control (or 'comparison') groups, enabling comparison of the processes and outcomes experienced within each.

sexual health Put positively, a state in which biological, psychological and/or social factors are such as to enable individuals to fulfill their potential in exercising choice and achieving contentment in their sexual identities and relationships. Put negatively, the absence of conditions that are either transmitted sexually, or which would hamper sexual relationships.

social and behavioural intervention Interventions that aim to influence how people interact or behave, by addressing factors such as knowledge, skills, views, and environment, using a variety of approaches such as education, counselling, and public policy.

systematic review A method whereby research reports are identified, collated, assessed and summarized in order to answer a pre-defined question using explicit and pre-specified methods and criteria.

Index